BARRON'S

PARAMEDIC
Exam

2ND EDITION

Mark Marchetta, RN, BS, NREMT-P
Director, EMS Education
Director, Trauma Services
Aultman Hospital
Canton, OH

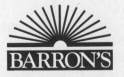

BARRON'S

DEDICATION

To my wife Loretta, the biggest supporter of my work.
Thank you for your tolerance, understanding, and sense of humor.

To my children Mark Jr. and Austin. You are truly the light of my life.
Thanks for making every day so precious.

To my parents who have supported me through all my endeavors.

All inquiries should be addressed to:
Barron's Educational Series, Inc.
250 Wireless Boulevard
Hauppauge, NY 11788
www.barronseduc.com

ISBN-13: 978-0-7641-9558-7 (book w/CD-ROM)
ISBN-10: 0-7641-9558-1 (book w/CD-ROM)

Library of Congress Catalog Card No. 2008018474

Library of Congress Cataloging-in-Publication Data
Marchetta, Mark.
    EMT-paramedic exam / Mark Marchetta.—2nd ed.
        p. ; cm.
    Rev. ed. of: How to prepare for the EMT-paramedic exam / Mark Marchetta. c2003.
    Includes index.
    ISBN-13: 978-0-7641-3939-0
    ISBN-10: 0-7641-3939-8
    ISBN-13: 978-0-7641-9558-7 (book w/CD-ROM)
    ISBN-10: 0-7641-9558-1 (book w/CD-ROM)
    1. Emergency medicine—United States—Examinations, questions, etc. 2. Emergency medical
technicians—Licences—United States—Study guides. I. Marchetta, Mark. How to prepare for the
EMT-paramedic exam. II. Title.
    [DNLM: 1. Emergencies—United States—Examination Questions. 2. Emergency Medical
Services—United States—Examination Questions. 3. Emergency Medical Technicians—United
States—Examination Questions. WB 18.2 M317e 2008]
    RC86.9.M367 2008
    616.02'5076—dc22
                                                                        2008018474

PRINTED IN THE UNITED STATES OF AMERICA
9 8 7 6 5 4 3 2 1

Contents

About the Author

M ark Marchetta has been involved in EMS for more than 21 years. He is an author, educator, and researcher. He has published 17 EMS research studies including a 2007 study on prehospital CPAP that has gained state, national, and international attention. He has served the state of Ohio since 1999 as a member of the State EMS Board and chairman of the State EMS Education Committee. He is also a member of the Advisory Board for the Prehospital Care Research Forum at UCLA Medical Center.

Contributors

arron's *Paramedic Exam* was written with the assistance of several educators who have demonstrated excellence in the clinical and classroom settings. The following individuals contributed to this book.

Patricia A. Ambrose, NREMT-P, CCEMT-P
EMS/Continuing Medical Education Coordinator
St. Vincent University of Toledo Medical Center
St. Rita's Life Flight/Mobile Life Critical Care Transport Network
Toledo, Ohio

K. A. Ballman, R.N., CEN, EMT-P
Bethesda Hospital
Cincinnati, Ohio

Alan F. Mistler, MEd, R.N., NREMT-P
University of Cincinnati
Cincinnati, Ohio

Chuck Sowerbrower, MEd, NCEE, NREMT-P
EMS Chairperson
Sinclair Community College
Dayton, Ohio

Brian Tritchler, B.S.N., R.N., CEN, EMT-P
Director, Paramedic Education
Summa Health System
Akron, Ohio

Medical Advisor:
Mike Mackan, MD, FACEP
Akron, Ohio

Manuscript Review:
Loretta L. Marchetta, R.N.
Hopedale, Ohio

Preface

The purpose of this book is to help you prepare for examinations in your Paramedic education course and for your state paramedic certification exam. If you are currently certified, this book will provide you with an effective review for a refresher or any recertification exam you may need to take.

The second edition of *Paramedic Exam* consists of multiple-choice questions accompanied by answers with the rationale. The material is based on information present in the current U.S. Department of Transportation National Standard EMT-Paramedic Curriculum and the Current National Registry of Emergency Medical Technicians Practice Analysis. Cardiology questions are based on the 2005 American Heart Association Guidelines for cardiac care.

This book consists of eight chapters. I strongly encourage you to start with Chapter One, "Tips for Preparing for and Taking the Test." You can then move to Chapters Two through Seven which contain exam questions. When reviewing the questions, it is important to have confidence choosing the correct answer. Confidence comes through understanding the material. If you find yourself missing several questions on one topic (e.g., management of seizures) or even if you get a question correct with a "lucky guess," it is essential you go back to the course material presented to you and make certain you *truly* understand the information. Memorizing the questions and answers to every question in this book will not ensure a passing grade on any examination. This book must be used as a tool to identify areas that require additional studying and understanding.

Once you review the questions and brush up on any material you may have found difficult, you can move to Chapter Eight of the book, which contains a practice test. The CD-ROM contains two additional practice exams. The CD-ROM exams will provide you with a different perspective of test taking. On the actual National Registry Exam, you are not allowed to skip questions or go back and change an answer. However, on the CD-ROM, in Practice Mode, you can mark a question, return to it later, and go back to previous questions. You will find that reading off a computer screen may fatigue you, especially if you are not accustomed to working on a computer. This will be great practice for preparing you for the National Registry Exam.

The practice tests will be a helpful assessment of how well you know the material. The practice tests are not divided into individual sections or chapters; instead, the questions are in no particular order. This random order mirrors the layout of the National Registry Exam.

This book will assist you in your studies and ultimately in passing your examination. Just remember, you have the luxury of thinking about what you are going to choose for your answer on your exam. When it actually comes to providing patient care, you must be able to call upon your education to assist you in decision making. That is why it's important to understand your course material and NOT memorize it.

Good luck in your EMS career.
Mark Marchetta

Tips for Preparing for and Taking the Test

This chapter contains essential information on test preparation including

- Studying for the test
- Preparation the day before the test
- Test-taking strategies
- Deciphering difficult information
- Information on the National Registry Exam
- Tips for taking a computer-adaptive test
- Advice for after the test

Ever wonder how some people can get all the answers on a test correct without ever studying? Are you one of those people or are you one of the others who get so anxious that you can't remember a thing?

"Most adults… get a bit stressed when they have an exam coming up. But it often hits adults harder than younger people. Children and teenagers take tests routinely in school, so test taking is a familiar part of their lives. But if you've been out of school for a while, you're less accustomed to being judged in this manner. You may also have more pressure to succeed on a test if you are taking it to obtain or advance a career."

The secret of being a good test taker isn't just in understanding the material. A big part of it has to do with attitude—How do you approach the test, with confidence or timidly like a scared little rabbit? Another part has to do with the following tips for preparing for and taking a test.

STUDYING FOR THE TEST

First—When will the test be given? Once you have that information, you can decide how much you are able to study and then fit studying into your already full schedule. Developing a plan to include study time in your day is very important. Starting early allows you to spend a little time studying each day.

Second—Find out what will be covered on the test, how many questions there will be, and how long you will have to take the exam. You're already off to a good start here—you've got a book that reviews the material that could be on the test. Talking with others who have taken the exam is another way to get an idea of what may be on the test. Just remember, questions vary from test to test and although the topics emphasized in this review manual may be similar, they will probably not be identical. Also, when talking with others, keep in mind that you are getting their perception of the test, which may not always be accurate.

Third —Make your study time as productive as possible. For most people, reading and reading leads to nothing more than a sore neck and a serious case of boredom. To make the material stick, your study needs to be as active as possible. The goal of active study is to engage as many areas of the brain as possible. One example of an active study method is called the triple-read system. It can be time-consuming but will yield great results. Here is how to use this system to improve your retention of information.

First, read the entire chapter. Your goal on the first read is to get the high points of the chapter. If you were reading a murder mystery, then the goal would be to remember who the killer was, who was murdered, the main characters, and where and when the story took place. But you should not focus on the fine details such as what type of knife was used or what the weather was. You will pick up this fine detail in the second read.

Now that you have the general flavor of the story, go back and read the entire chapter a second time. This time focus on details. Look more closely at tables and graphs. Make sure you have looked up any concepts that are confusing. Focus on new words. Make sure that at the conclusion of this read, you understand all the concepts within the chapter.

The third read has the goal of creating an outline of the chapter. Go back and read the entire chapter a third time. As you read, create an outline. This allows you to distill the large amount of information into something more manageable. This also provides you with a product that you can use for study.

Performing the triple-read method on the entire paramedic curriculum may not be possible because it is time-consuming. However, it is an effective study tool and should be used on material you find difficult. As you go through this study manual, if you find yourself missing questions on a particular topic over and over, you should certainly review that material prior to the test.

Other techniques that can turn passive study into a more active process include:

1. Rewrite your class notes.
2. Create flash cards.
3. Write mock test questions.
4. If you have tape-recorded the class, transcribe the recording.
5. Work in study groups and quiz each other on material.

Use your imagination. The goal of active study is to engage as many parts of your brain as possible. Ever forget the details about a concept but remember where on a page you wrote the notes? That is because in addition to a hearing and seeing memory, you also have the memory of writing the note (kinesthetic memory).

Fourth—Elicit support from your family. Studying will probably affect your family in some way. It may take time away from activities, you may need quiet time, or you may need a quiet place, all of which may be very difficult in a typical family. Your family needs to understand the importance of the test so they can understand your schedule and give you the support and encouragement you need.

THE DAY BEFORE THE TEST

Conduct a final review. This is not the time to try to learn new material—this should truly be a review.

Get a good night's rest. It is important to be well rested before a big test. It is easier to think when you are rested. Studies show that we can function on very little sleep, but that activities are not performed at the highest level of mental functioning. It will be harder to pull the information from the crevices of your brain, and you don't want that to happen during the test.

Make sure you know where to go to take the test. If the location is unfamiliar, it is probably a good idea to take a "trial run" and find the testing site. Getting lost on your way to the test can be frustrating and will significantly raise your stress level.

Get all your materials and supplies ready. For some tests you need a special admission card or form of identification. Do you need a #2 pencil? If so, make sure you have an adequate supply that are sharpened and have erasers. Some people like to take a supply of hard candies to help them stay awake, and if you are one of those people, make sure that this is allowed. For the National Registry Exam you will need photo identification.

Plan to arrive a few minutes early on the day of the test. There may be problems on the way to the test site—such as a traffic jam or car trouble. It also gives you time to relax, go to the bathroom, get a drink, and so on. Talk with others but avoid discussions of what they have studied or think will be on the test, as this can lead to test anxiety.

TEST-TAKING STRATEGIES

1. Use the 3 R's of good test taking. Read, Respond, and Relax.

   Read. Make sure that you read the entire question and each of the options. Many of the questions you will be answering will require you to gather and understand the details within the question. A blood pressure of 120/80 and one of 120/40 is NOT the same. Your goal is to understand the environment the question is creating. If you are finding yourself saying, "I would do different things in different circumstances," then you have probably missed the point of the question. Reread, again for detail.

   Respond. Once you have read the entire question and each option, then respond. Choose the answer that appears to be correct. If you are sure you have read the question and have gathered all the information and you remain unsure how to answer, then guess. Do not sit there and struggle if you have no idea how to respond. Simply choose an option and move on. Go with your first instinct.

   Relax. Arguably the hardest of the 3 R's is to remember to take time to clear your head. Envision the test as a marathon, not a sprint. You should not speed your way through just because you are a fast reader. Take your time, read the questions, and think about the answers. Every 30–40 questions, take a moment to close your eyes and shut the test out of your mind. Think of something that relaxes you. This will allow you to remain focused.

2. Read each question *and* all the options carefully. Look for words that may alter the meaning, e.g., always, never, usually, most, except, primary, most important. Often they are highlighted in some way to make them more noticeable. Remember to answer the question that is being asked. If the question asks you to choose the most important option, that does not imply that the other options are not important. All it means is that one option has more weight than the others.

DECIPHERING DIFFICULT INFORMATION

Scenario: A 45-year-old male patient states that he is having "severe chest pain." The pain started 20 minutes ago and has been increasing in intensity. He is complaining of nausea and shortness of breath. His skin is pale, cool, and clammy. Vital signs are blood pressure 112/86, pulse 110, respirations 20. What is your highest priority with this patient?

One approach to understanding complex questions is to determine what is known, what is implied, and what is assumed. In this three-level system, your goal is to focus only on the first two levels, known and implied. Look at the example.

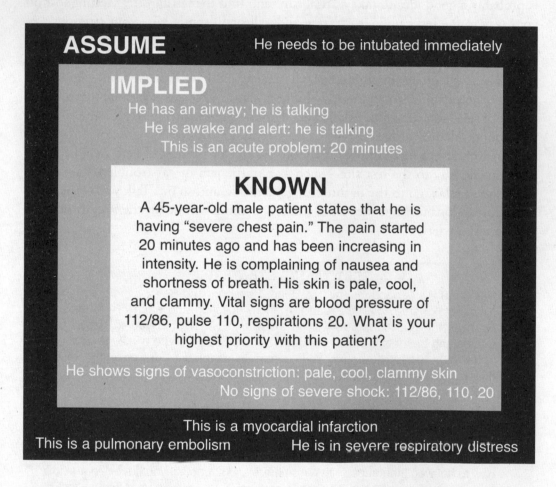

The inner box in white holds all the information from the question. This information is known and is true. The next box out, in light gray, holds all the information that MUST be true to make the inner box true. For example, a talking patient must have a pulse, have an airway, be moving air, have enough blood pressure to allow his brain to operate, and so on. These two levels are the extent to which any student is expected to go. The final outer level is assumed information, and we all know what happens when we assume.

In the outer (assumed) level, you are required to "what if" the question. You now need to take two steps away from the base information, and that is too far. At this level, you must assume or speculate. From the given information many possibilities present themselves. This is the level at which the test taker is "reading into the question." If you find yourself saying, "If this were an MI, I would do (B). But if this patient were in respiratory distress, I would do (C)" then you have missed the intent of the question. Go back, reread, and take only ONE STEP away from the given information.

The goal of this question deciphering is to discover what the author of the question is saying without saying it. The secondary goal is to prevent the test taker from reading into the question.

NATIONAL REGISTRY EXAM

When taking the National Registry computer-based examination there are some important differences that you need to be aware of. This is a high-stakes test. People are trying to get jobs based on the results of this test, so security is high to ensure all testing candidates are equally evaluated. When you arrive, you will be asked to remove all telecommunication/electronic devices. A locker will be assigned to you for your cell phone, purse, jacket, and so on. You may even be pat-searched before you are allowed to enter the testing area.

While testing, you will be constantly monitored. You will not be able to move about the testing area without permission. Do not allow this strict security to unnerve you. The intent is to ensure that all candidates are tested on their knowledge level.

While taking the computer-based exam, you will not be permitted to skip questions. Once you are presented with a question, the computer will wait until you answer to continue. It is also important to keep in mind that this is a timed test. Remaining on one question for a long period of time is not advisable.

On January 1, 2007, National Registry testing changed to computer-adaptive testing (CAT). This type of testing adapts to each student. The computer uses a specialized program to determine whether or not the student has enough knowledge to pass the test. The computer knows the difficulty of each question. Based on how well you respond to a question, the computer then chooses another question. If you got an easy question correct, the computer will choose a more difficult one. If you got a difficult question wrong, a slightly easier one is chosen. This process continues until the computer is relatively certain whether or not you have enough knowledge to pass the test.

Let's use an analogy to help understand CAT. Imagine you are standing in a darkened room. There is no light, you are completely hidden from view, and the computer is trying to see you.

After you answer each question, the computer shines a small light to see you. The number of questions correct or incorrect determines "how" the computer sees you. It keeps doing this until enough lights are shining on whether you passed or whether you failed. The more consistent you are with your answers, the more quickly the computer can come to a conclusion. Most students will complete the test in 70–100 questions. This means that your answers were consistent: either consistently right or consistently wrong.

The computer needs to be 95% certain on the results, so some students need more questions than others. An increased number of questions indicates the computer is having trouble finding you within the room. Do not panic! The computer has not determined a passing or failing score. Keep calm and answer the questions correctly. You are deep into the test, and a passing score is just a few correct answers away!

The implications of CAT are that no two students will ever have the exact same test. Another consequence of this style of testing is that a record of each question you have seen is kept. This means that if you need to be tested a second time, you will never see the same questions again. The computer will simply choose another question from the test bank.

TIPS FOR TAKING A COMPUTER-ADAPTIVE TEST

1. Be prepared for a high-security environment. No one is accusing you of cheating. The system wants to ensure all candidates have the same opportunities to be successful.
2. You will not be able to go back and change answers, so read each question thoroughly. If you have no idea what the answer is, guess and move on.
3. The questions will be predominately scenario based.
4. There will be very few questions that have, all of the above, none of the above, except, never, always, and so on.
5. There will be many questions that require you to prioritize or choose between options that are close.
6. Do not answer questions based solely on protocols. "Airway is always first" will not get you through the test. You must understand the question clearly and then respond. If you can answer the question solely by looking at the options, then you are probably wrong.
7. Monitor the number of questions you are answering. A display will tell you what question number you are on. If you find yourself at question 100, this may indicate inconsistency in your responses. The best course of action is to slow down and ensure that you have read the question clearly.

ADVICE FOR AFTER THE TEST

It is not a good idea to talk about the test with the other test takers. This tends to increase your anxiety, especially if you find they have answered questions differently. The test is over and you cannot go back and change any of your answers. Besides— everyone's perception of the test—hard or easy—and what they remember will be different based on what they studied and what their own personal strengths and weaknesses are. You have made it this far—the worst is over—all you can do now is wait for the results! Reward yourself for making it through the test—you (and your family) deserve to spend some time on something fun for a change.

Airway and Breathing

 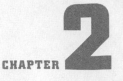

This chapter contains questions on airway and breathing assessment, proper interventions for patients with respiratory compromise, oxygen delivery systems, ventilatory support, and respiratory anatomy and physiology.

There are also questions on basic airway management and basic cardiopulmonary resuscitation. Give these questions due consideration because *it is a fact* that you must do *basic* interventions before you can perform *advanced* interventions.

It is common for paramedic students to answer basic airway and breathing questions incorrectly because they want to go directly to the advanced interventions. Don't fall into this trap!

Answer Sheet

CHAPTER 2—AIRWAY AND BREATHING

1 Ⓐ Ⓑ Ⓒ Ⓓ	21 Ⓐ Ⓑ Ⓒ Ⓓ	41 Ⓐ Ⓑ Ⓒ Ⓓ	61 Ⓐ Ⓑ Ⓒ Ⓓ
2 Ⓐ Ⓑ Ⓒ Ⓓ	22 Ⓐ Ⓑ Ⓒ Ⓓ	42 Ⓐ Ⓑ Ⓒ Ⓓ	62 Ⓐ Ⓑ Ⓒ Ⓓ
3 Ⓐ Ⓑ Ⓒ Ⓓ	23 Ⓐ Ⓑ Ⓒ Ⓓ	43 Ⓐ Ⓑ Ⓒ Ⓓ	63 Ⓐ Ⓑ Ⓒ Ⓓ
4 Ⓐ Ⓑ Ⓒ Ⓓ	24 Ⓐ Ⓑ Ⓒ Ⓓ	44 Ⓐ Ⓑ Ⓒ Ⓓ	64 Ⓐ Ⓑ Ⓒ Ⓓ
5 Ⓐ Ⓑ Ⓒ Ⓓ	25 Ⓐ Ⓑ Ⓒ Ⓓ	45 Ⓐ Ⓑ Ⓒ Ⓓ	65 Ⓐ Ⓑ Ⓒ Ⓓ
6 Ⓐ Ⓑ Ⓒ Ⓓ	26 Ⓐ Ⓑ Ⓒ Ⓓ	46 Ⓐ Ⓑ Ⓒ Ⓓ	66 Ⓐ Ⓑ Ⓒ Ⓓ
7 Ⓐ Ⓑ Ⓒ Ⓓ	27 Ⓐ Ⓑ Ⓒ Ⓓ	47 Ⓐ Ⓑ Ⓒ Ⓓ	67 Ⓐ Ⓑ Ⓒ Ⓓ
8 Ⓐ Ⓑ Ⓒ Ⓓ	28 Ⓐ Ⓑ Ⓒ Ⓓ	48 Ⓐ Ⓑ Ⓒ Ⓓ	68 Ⓐ Ⓑ Ⓒ Ⓓ
9 Ⓐ Ⓑ Ⓒ Ⓓ	29 Ⓐ Ⓑ Ⓒ Ⓓ	49 Ⓐ Ⓑ Ⓒ Ⓓ	69 Ⓐ Ⓑ Ⓒ Ⓓ
10 Ⓐ Ⓑ Ⓒ Ⓓ	30 Ⓐ Ⓑ Ⓒ Ⓓ	50 Ⓐ Ⓑ Ⓒ Ⓓ	70 Ⓐ Ⓑ Ⓒ Ⓓ
11 Ⓐ Ⓑ Ⓒ Ⓓ	31 Ⓐ Ⓑ Ⓒ Ⓓ	51 Ⓐ Ⓑ Ⓒ Ⓓ	71 Ⓐ Ⓑ Ⓒ Ⓓ
12 Ⓐ Ⓑ Ⓒ Ⓓ	32 Ⓐ Ⓑ Ⓒ Ⓓ	52 Ⓐ Ⓑ Ⓒ Ⓓ	72 Ⓐ Ⓑ Ⓒ Ⓓ
13 Ⓐ Ⓑ Ⓒ Ⓓ	33 Ⓐ Ⓑ Ⓒ Ⓓ	53 Ⓐ Ⓑ Ⓒ Ⓓ	73 Ⓐ Ⓑ Ⓒ Ⓓ
14 Ⓐ Ⓑ Ⓒ Ⓓ	34 Ⓐ Ⓑ Ⓒ Ⓓ	54 Ⓐ Ⓑ Ⓒ Ⓓ	74 Ⓐ Ⓑ Ⓒ Ⓓ
15 Ⓐ Ⓑ Ⓒ Ⓓ	35 Ⓐ Ⓑ Ⓒ Ⓓ	55 Ⓐ Ⓑ Ⓒ Ⓓ	75 Ⓐ Ⓑ Ⓒ Ⓓ
16 Ⓐ Ⓑ Ⓒ Ⓓ	36 Ⓐ Ⓑ Ⓒ Ⓓ	56 Ⓐ Ⓑ Ⓒ Ⓓ	76 Ⓐ Ⓑ Ⓒ Ⓓ
17 Ⓐ Ⓑ Ⓒ Ⓓ	37 Ⓐ Ⓑ Ⓒ Ⓓ	57 Ⓐ Ⓑ Ⓒ Ⓓ	77 Ⓐ Ⓑ Ⓒ Ⓓ
18 Ⓐ Ⓑ Ⓒ Ⓓ	38 Ⓐ Ⓑ Ⓒ Ⓓ	58 Ⓐ Ⓑ Ⓒ Ⓓ	78 Ⓐ Ⓑ Ⓒ Ⓓ
19 Ⓐ Ⓑ Ⓒ Ⓓ	39 Ⓐ Ⓑ Ⓒ Ⓓ	59 Ⓐ Ⓑ Ⓒ Ⓓ	79 Ⓐ Ⓑ Ⓒ Ⓓ
20 Ⓐ Ⓑ Ⓒ Ⓓ	40 Ⓐ Ⓑ Ⓒ Ⓓ	60 Ⓐ Ⓑ Ⓒ Ⓓ	80 Ⓐ Ⓑ Ⓒ Ⓓ

1. A child in respiratory distress may grunt as the child breathes. This is
   a result of
   (A) increasing tidal volume.
   (B) an increased respiratory rate.
   (C) creating pressure to help maintain open airways.
   (D) an indication that the child is tired and will progress to respiratory
   arrest.

2. Respiratory acidosis is caused by
   (A) an excess of bicarbonate.
   (B) excess carbon dioxide retention.
   (C) a loss of bicarbonate.
   (D) excess carbon dioxide excretion.

Questions 3 and 4 are based on the following scenario:

You are using an end-tidal carbon dioxide detector as a tool to assist for proper
endotracheal intubation placement.

3. The absence of carbon dioxide in exhaled air indicates the endotracheal tube
   has been
   (A) placed in the right mainstem bronchus.
   (B) correctly placed in the trachea.
   (C) placed in the esophagus.
   (D) placed in the left mainstem bronchus.

4. Your next action is to
   (A) deflate the cuff, pull the endotracheal tube back 2 cm, and reassess
   placement.
   (B) secure the endotracheal tube and confirm correct placement by auscultation.
   (C) inflate the distal cuff with 7–10 cc of air and secure the endotracheal
   tube.
   (D) remove the endotracheal tube and provide several ventilations prior to
   attempting intubation again.

---

5. Which of the following drugs is used for rapid sequence intubation?

   (A) Vecuronium
   (B) Succinylcholine
   (C) Lidocaine and atropine
   (D) All of the above

6. You are called for a 54-year-old woman who is unconscious. Your assessment reveals the patient to be apneic and pulseless. Initial management of this patient's airway should include
   (A) assisted ventilation with a bag-valve device at 6–10 LPM.
   (B) assisted ventilation with a nonrebreather mask at 10–15 LPM.
   (C) immediate nasotracheal intubation and ventilation with a bag-valve device.
   (D) insertion of an oropharyngeal airway and ventilation with a bag-valve device.

7. The Esophageal Tracheal Combitube (ETCT) and the pharyngotracheal lumen airway (PTL) are similar because
   (A) neither requires assessment for accurate placement.
   (B) both require manipulation of the head and neck for insertion.
   (C) neither is inserted blindly.
   (D) None of the above.

8. Breath sounds such as crackles and rhonchi that are not normally heard are defined as _____ breath sounds.
   (A) bronchial
   (B) adventitious
   (C) vesicular
   (D) bronchovesicular

9. Which of the following correctly describes the flow of air from outside the body into the trachea?
   (A) Nose, nasopharynx, laryngopharynx, oropharynx, larynx, trachea
   (B) Nose, nasopharynx, larynx, laryngopharynx, oropharynx, trachea
   (C) Nose, nasal cavities, nasopharynx, oropharynx, laryngopharynx, larynx, trachea
   (D) Nose, nasal cavities, laryngopharynx, nasopharynx, oropharynx, larynx, trachea

10. You are called for an unresponsive 29-year-old man. Bystanders report he has been drinking heavily all day. Assessment reveals the patient to be responsive only to painful stimuli. His breathing is shallow at a rate of four times per minute. How would you manage this patient?
    (A) Nasal cannula at 2–4 LPM
    (B) Simple face mask at 4–6 LPM
    (C) Nonrebreather mask at 10–15 LPM
    (D) Bag-valve device with a reservoir at 10–15 LPM

11. The normal arterial pH range in the human body is
    (A) 7.0–7.15
    (B) 7.15–7.35
    (C) 7.35–7.45
    (D) 7.45–7.80

12. You have orally intubated a patient. While your partner ventilates the patient with a bag-valve device, you assess for proper placement. Auscultation reveals sounds heard over the right chest and an absence of breath sounds over the left chest. Your best course of action would be to
    (A) hyperventilate the patient and prepare the equipment necessary for a surgical cricothyrotomy.
    (B) deflate the endotracheal tube cuff, withdraw the tube 2 cm and reevaluate breath sounds, and reinflate the cuff.
    (C) deflate the endotracheal tube cuff, remove the endotracheal tube, and hyperventilate the patient with a bag-valve device.
    (D) insert a large diameter needle into the fourth or fifth intercostal space, midaxillary line.

13. The Sellick maneuver
    (A) is used to clear a foreign body airway obstruction in an infant or child.
    (B) is used to clear blood or mucus from an endotracheal tube or the nasopharynx.
    (C) may be used to minimize gastric distention and facilitate placement of an endotracheal tube into the glottic opening.
    (D) is the preferred method for opening the airway of an unconscious patient when cervical spine injury is suspected.

14. The area where the trachea divides into the right and left mainstem bronchi is known as the
    (A) pleura.
    (B) xiphoid process.
    (C) carina.
    (D) sternal angle.

15. The administration of which of the following may result in a decrease in the respiratory rate?
    (A) Nubain
    (B) Diltiazem
    (C) Cordarone
    (D) Morphine sulphate

16. The anatomical structure between the base of the tongue and the epiglottis into which the tip of the curved blade (Macintosh blade) is placed during orotracheal intubation is the
    (A) carina.
    (B) vallecula.
    (C) glottis.
    (D) esophagus.

17. The term used to describe normal breath sounds heard over most of the chest wall is
    (A) bronchial.
    (B) adventitious.
    (C) vesicular.
    (D) bronchovesicular.

18. When blood levels of carbon dioxide or hydrogen ions increase above normal, the respiratory center of the brain responds by
    (A) decreasing the rate and increasing the depth of respiration.
    (B) increasing the rate and depth of respiration.
    (C) increasing the rate and decreasing the depth of respiration.
    (D) decreasing the rate and decreasing the depth of respiration.

19. The blood component responsible for transporting oxygen from the lungs to the body tissues and transporting carbon dioxide from the body tissues to the lungs is the
    (A) plasma.
    (B) platelets.
    (C) leukocytes.
    (D) erythrocytes.

20. Which of the following is an advantage of the laryngeal mask airway (LMA)?
    (A) It is blindly inserted.
    (B) It isolates the esophagus.
    (C) It does not protect against regurgitation and aspiration.
    (D) It can be used with an intact gag reflex.

21. You have a female patient with a long history of COPD who complains of worsening shortness of breath. She is on continuous 2 LPM of home oxygen. You are concerned that increasing the oxygen flow may eliminate the hypoxic drive to breathe because the hypoxic drive is regulated by
    (A) high PaO_2.
    (B) low PaO_2.
    (C) high oxygen saturation.
    (D) low oxygen saturation.

22. You arrive on the scene of a patient who is receiving bag-valve-mask ventilation. The abdomen is extremely distended. After intubation, you have resistance while bagging the patient. Lung sounds are diminished bilaterally, and the trachea is midline. What should you do?
    (A) Suction for foreign body aspiration.
    (B) Insert a naso/oral gastric tube.
    (C) Pull back the ET tube 2 cm and reassess.
    (D) Reassess for development of pneumothorax.

23. The simplest airway management technique in a patient *without* suspected cervical spine injury is
    (A) head-tilt/chin-lift maneuver.
    (B) modified jaw-thrust maneuver.
    (C) endotracheal intubation.
    (D) nasotracheal intubation.

24. The proper size oropharyngeal airway is determined by measuring
    (A) from the tip of the nose to the center of the chin.
    (B) from the corner of the mouth to the tip of the chin.
    (C) from the corner of the mouth to the tip of the earlobe at the angle of the jaw.
    (D) from the center of the mouth to the tip of the earlobe at the angle of the jaw.

25. The normal value for PCO_2 is
    (A) 7.00 to 7.15.
    (B) 22 to 26 mEq/liter.
    (C) 35 to 45 mmHg.
    (D) 80 to 100 mmHg.

26. The maximum water pressure recommended for positive pressure ventilation should not exceed_____ cm.
    (A) 15
    (B) 30
    (C) 50
    (D) 60

27. Manual maneuvers used to open a patient's airway
    (A) are contraindicated in most patients.
    (B) are difficult to perform.
    (C) include head tilt/chin lift and jaw thrust.
    (D) do not usually work without more extensive intervention.

28. The major advantage of the use of CPAP and BiPAP devices is
    (A) intubation may be avoided.
    (B) there are no contraindications for their use.
    (C) they can be used in an apneic patient.
    (D) all of the above.

29. Digital intubation may be helpful when:
    (A) there is suspected spinal cord injury.
    (B) the tongue is swollen.
    (C) the respiratory rate is 4/minute.
    (D) upper airway obstruction is suspected.

30. Advantages of the Esophageal Tracheal CombiTube include all of the following except
    (A) insertion is rapid and easy.
    (B) it can be used on trauma patients.
    (C) it can provide ventilation if placed in the esophagus.
    (D) it can be used with pediatric patients.

31. Causes for decreased $ETCO_2$ readings include
    (A) nonperfusing patient.
    (B) presence of severe acidosis.
    (C) presence of pulmonary emboli.
    (D) all of the above.

Questions 32 and 33 are based on the following scenario:

You are caring for a male patient in ventricular tachycardia. He is lethargic, diaphoretic, pale, and has vomited once. His vital signs are: BP 74/P, pulse 184, respirations 14. You are assigned to manage the airway.

32. Initial management should include
    (A) high-flow oxygen by nonrebreather mask.
    (B) preparation for intubation.
    (C) bag-valve mask ventilations.
    (D) suctioning the airway for vomitus.

33. Your patient becomes unresponsive and apneic. Further airway management should include
    (A) providing ventilations through a nonrebreather mask.
    (B) bag-valve mask ventilation at 20 times per minute.
    (C) endotracheal intubation.
    (D) oral airway insertion and supplemental oxygen by nonrebreather mask.

---

34. Succinylcholine is contraindicated in patients with crush injuries because of

    (A) hypovolemia.
    (B) risk of hyperkalemia.
    (C) increased muscle tremors.
    (D) risk of laryngeal edema.

35. What effects does hyperventilation have on cerebral circulation and intracranial pressure?
    (A) More pronounced decrease in circulation than decrease in intracranial pressure
    (B) Vasoconstriction and increased intracranial pressure
    (C) Vasodilation and decreased intracranial pressure
    (D) Little or no effect on cerebral circulation or intracranial pressure

36. You arrive at the scene of an accident in which a car has struck a telephone pole. You find a 17-year-old female ejected from her vehicle, lying 25 feet from the point of impact. Which of the following is an acceptable method of opening her airway?
    (A) Jaw thrust
    (B) Neck extension
    (C) Neck flexion
    (D) Sellick's maneuver

37. Which of the following is not considered a sign or symptom indicating a tension pneumothorax?
    (A) Dyspnea
    (B) Hyperresonance to percussion
    (C) Distended jugular veins
    (D) Clear lung sounds

38. After decompressing the chest of the victim with a tension pneumothorax, you determine your intervention was successful by observing for
    (A) air rushing from the catheter.
    (B) a decrease in the patient's cyanosis.
    (C) an improvement in the patient's level of consciousness.
    (D) an improvement in the patient's ventilatory and circulatory status.

39. During needle decompression, the needle is inserted on the top of the rib for what purpose?
    (A) To ensure that the vein, artery, and nerve bundle under each rib are not damaged
    (B) To ensure proper placement
    (C) To ensure that the catheter enters the pleural space at the correct angle
    (D) To ensure that the site does not become a sucking chest wound

40. You have intubated a patient with a long history of chronic bronchitis. During transport, you notice that ventilations are becoming increasingly difficult. You auscultate the chest and hear faint equal breath sounds. What intervention is most likely indicated for this patient?
    (A) Increasing ventilation rate to 16/minute
    (B) Withdrawing the ET tube 2 cm and reassessing
    (C) Tracheobronchial suctioning
    (D) Gastric decompression

41. A drop in systolic blood pressure of 10 mmHg or more or the absence of a radial pulse during inspiration is known as
    (A) pericardial tamponade.
    (B) pulsus paradoxus.
    (C) orthostatic change.
    (D) pulse pressure change.

42. A nasal cannula will deliver ___ % of oxygen at a flow rate of 6 LPM in optimal conditions.
    (A) 30
    (B) 40
    (C) 50
    (D) 65

43. A nonrebreather mask can deliver an oxygen concentration of _____% at a flow rate of 15 LPM.
    (A) 40 to 60
    (B) 60 to 80
    (C) 80 to 95
    (D) 90 to 100

44. A bag-valve mask device with a reservoir and an adequate oxygen source (at least 15 LPM) will deliver an oxygen concentration of
    (A) 21%.
    (B) 40% to 60%.
    (C) 80%.
    (D) 100%.

45. The minimum size bag-valve mask device used for neonates, infants, and children should be
    (A) 250 ml.
    (B) 450 ml.
    (C) 750 ml.
    (D) 1,000 ml.

46. You respond to a 72-year-old man with syncope. He is sitting in the kitchen when you arrive. He is alert and oriented to person, place, and time. He complains of dizziness. Current vitals are BP 108/60, pulse 96 slightly irregular, and respirations of 28. Pulse oximeter reading is 97%. ECG shows a sinus rhythm with occasional PVC's. This patient should receive oxygen
    (A) by nasal cannula at 3 LPM.
    (B) by nonrebreather mask.
    (C) oxygen application is not required.
    (D) by nasal cannula at 6 LPM.

47. Suctioning (application of negative pressure) should be activated
    (A) upon insertion of the suction catheter.
    (B) upon extraction of the suction catheter.
    (C) both upon insertion and extraction.
    (D) either upon insertion or extraction (it makes no difference).

48. The nasopharyngeal airway should be measured
    (A) from the corner of the mouth to the earlobe.
    (B) from the tip of the nose to the earlobe.
    (C) from the tip of the nose to the corner of the mouth.
    (D) from the tip of the nose to the chin.

49. When using a straight blade (Miller blade) to intubate an adult patient, the tip of the blade should be placed
    (A) directly on or under the epiglottis.
    (B) above the epiglottis.
    (C) in the vallecula.
    (D) past the epiglottis at the vocal cords.

50. When intubating an adult patient with a curved blade (Macintosh blade), the tip of the blade should be placed
    (A) under the epiglottis.
    (B) in the vallecula, at the base of the tongue.
    (C) in the vallecula, at the opening of the vocal cords.
    (D) to the right of the epiglottis.

51. When confirming endotracheal tube placement, it is imperative to auscultate
    (A) at the midaxillary line.
    (B) over the trachea.
    (C) over the epigastrium.
    (D) All of the above.

52. A respiratory pattern characterized by a gradually increasing rate and tidal volume followed by a gradual decrease with intermittent periods of apnea is
    (A) Cheyne-Stokes.
    (B) Biot's (ataxic).
    (C) central neurogenic hyperventilation.
    (D) agonal.

53. A respiratory pattern characterized by an irregular pattern, rate, and volume with intermittent periods of apnea is
    (A) Cheyne-Stokes.
    (B) Biot's (ataxic).
    (C) central neurogenic hyperventilation.
    (D) agonal.

54. A respiratory pattern characterized by deep, rapid respirations is
    (A) Cheyne-Stokes.
    (B) Biot's (ataxic).
    (C) central neurogenic hyperventilation.
    (D) agonal.

55. A respiratory pattern characterized by slow, shallow, irregular respirations is
    (A) Cheyne-Stokes.
    (B) Biot's (ataxic).
    (C) central neurogenic hyperventilation.
    (D) bradypnea.

56. All of the following can affect the accuracy reading of a pulse oximeter except
    (A) hypoperfusion.
    (B) anemia.
    (C) carbon monoxide poisoning.
    (D) hyperthermia.

57. Complications of endotracheal intubation include all of the following except
    (A) trauma to the teeth.
    (B) gastric distension.
    (C) esophageal intubation.
    (D) laryngospasm.

58. Confirmation of endotracheal tube placement should be evaluated
    (A) immediately after insertion.
    (B) each time the patient is moved.
    (C) by at least two methods.
    (D) All of the above.

59. A high-pitched noise associated with upper airway constriction is known as
    (A) wheezing.
    (B) rhonchi.
    (C) stridor.
    (D) rales.

60. Before providing rescue breathing to an unresponsive victim, you must check for breathing. You do this by
    (A) opening the airway.
    (B) shaking and shouting to stimulate the victim to breathe.
    (C) looking, listening, and feeling airflow through the victim's nose or mouth.
    (D) establishing unresponsiveness.

61. You are performing rescue breathing on an adult. How many breaths do you give?
    (A) One breath every 12 seconds
    (B) One breath every 5 seconds
    (C) Two breaths every 10 seconds
    (D) Two breaths every 6 seconds

62. Where should you place your hands on the chest of an adult victim when you are performing chest compressions?
    (A) On the upper half of the sternum
    (B) On the lower one third of the sternum
    (C) On the lower half of the sternum, at the nipple line
    (D) Over the very bottom of the sternum

63. What is the ratio of compressions to ventilations when performing one-person CPR on an adult?
    (A) 5 compressions to 1 ventilation
    (B) 30 compressions to 1 ventilation
    (C) 30 compressions to 2 ventilations
    (D) 15 compressions to 2 ventilations

64. What is the correct rate you should use to perform chest compressions for an adult victim of cardiac arrest?
    (A) 100 times per minute
    (B) 60 times per minute
    (C) 120 times per minute
    (D) 80 times per minute

65. You are performing rescue breathing with a bag-mask device for an apneic child. How often should you provide rescue breaths?
    (A) Once every 3 seconds
    (B) Once every 6 seconds
    (C) Once every 9 seconds
    (D) Twice every 6 seconds

66. You are caring for a 77-year-old male patient who is short of breath and has a history of COPD. He is alert and oriented to person, place, and time but able to speak only in two- to three-word sentences. What does the patient's ability to speak in two- to three-word sentences indicate?
    (A) Respiratory alkalosis is present.
    (B) Inadequate tidal volume is present.
    (C) His condition is improving.
    (D) Respiratory acidosis is present.

67. You observe a COPD patient utilizing the pursed-lip breathing technique. Which statement is correct regarding pursed-lip breathing?
    (A) It is not usually used by COPD patients.
    (B) It may eliminate the hypoxic drive to breath.
    (C) It helps improve tidal volume.
    (D) It helps maintain pressure within the airways.

68. In a patient in respiratory distress, the development of which sign/symptom would lead you to believe the patient is significantly decompensating?
    (A) Decreased level of consciousness
    (B) JVD
    (C) Cyanosis
    (D) Increase in blood pressure

69. You respond to a cafeteria for a 16-year-old patient who is choking. Your patient is conscious and coughing forcefully. She appears anxious and is difficult to communicate with due to the coughing but is able to follow commands. Assessment reveals a respiratory rate of 28, shallow, diminished breath sounds on the right side, and a SpO_2 reading of 96%. Based on the history and assessment findings, you suspect
    (A) aspiration of food into the right mainstem bronchus causing obstruction.
    (B) a spontaneous pneumothorax on the left side secondary to the forceful coughing.
    (C) that the choking episode has subsided and the patient is recovering.
    (D) a spontaneous pneumothorax on the right side secondary to the forceful coughing.

70. Nasotracheal intubation is contraindicated in a patient with
    (A) clenched teeth.
    (B) a history of recent sinus infections.
    (C) a suspected basilar skull fracture.
    (D) facial trauma.

71. Blind nasotracheal intubation
    (A) should be attempted only on an apneic patient.
    (B) is preferred over oral intubation.
    (C) should be attempted on a patient with spontaneous respirations.
    (D) is contraindicated when facial trauma is present.

72. An infant should not be suctioned for more than
    (A) 15 seconds.
    (B) 5 seconds.
    (C) 10 seconds.
    (D) 20 seconds.

73. One reason the respiratory system of a geriatric patient becomes less effective is that
    (A) the muscles of the diaphragm weaken.
    (B) tidal volume increases.
    (C) there is decreased chest wall compliance.
    (D) the lungs become more compliant.

74. You respond to the home of a 17-year-old male because his father was unable to wake him. The father states that his son was at a party last night and has a history of recreational drug use. He is unconscious and unresponsive. BP is not obtainable, pulse 42 and weak, and respirations of 4. You have orally intubated the patient. Auscultation of lung sounds post intubation reveal breath sounds heard over the right chest and an absence of breath sounds over the left chest. Your next action would be to
    (A) hyperventilate the patient and reassess lung sounds.
    (B) deflate the endotracheal tube cuff, withdraw the tube 2 cm and reevaluate breath sounds, and reinflate the cuff.
    (C) deflate the endotracheal tube cuff, remove the endotracheal tube, and hyperventilate the patient with a bag-valve device.
    (D) observe the patient and monitor his SpO_2 reading for several minutes.

75. All of the following are reasons for a pulse oximeter to read "Error" except
    (A) low capillary blood flow.
    (B) peripheral vasoconstriction.
    (C) extremity movement.
    (D) hyperthermia.

76. Field extubation is indicated if the patient
    (A) is awake and able to maintain his or her own airway.
    (B) is unconscious and continually bites the endotracheal tube.
    (C) is not suspected of alcohol intoxication.
    (D) becomes combative and starts to delay additional treatment.

77. You have successfully resuscitated a patient who suffered a cardiac arrest. You are enroute to the hospital when the patient wakes up and is not tolerating the endotracheal tube. The medical director at the receiving hospital has ordered you to extubate the patient. All of the following should be done except
    (A) removing the endotracheal tube on a cough or expiration.
    (B) deflating the endotracheal tube cuff completely.
    (C) removing the endotracheal tube slowly.
    (D) providing supplemental oxygen once the tube is removed.

78. You arrive on the scene of a 40-year-old male with a complaint of palpations and dizziness. Vitals are BP 102/78, pulse 128 slightly irregular, and respirations of 26. A pulse oximeter reading of 86% is obtained. He has no past medical problems. With this information, you suspect
    (A) hyperventilation syndrome.
    (B) hypoxemia.
    (C) congestive heart failure.
    (D) pending respiratory arrest.

79. The presence of rhonchi in a patient diagnosed with pneumonia indicates
    (A) narrowing of the airways.
    (B) a normal finding in a pneumonia patient.
    (C) onset of bronchitis.
    (D) mucus in the airways.

80. When using a bulb syringe device to assist in verification of proper endotracheal tube placement, all of the following are true except
    (A) if the bulb syringe easily inflates, the endotracheal tube is correctly placed in the trachea.
    (B) if the bulb syringe does not inflate, the endotracheal tube is placed in the esophagus.
    (C) the cuff on the endotracheal tube must be inflated prior to using a bulb syringe device.
    (D) the cuff on the endotracheal tube should not be inflated prior to using a bulb syringe device.

ANSWERS AND ANSWER EXPLANATIONS

1. **(C)** Grunting involves exhaling against a partially closed glottis. This creates pressure to help maintain open lower airways similar to pursed-lip breathing in adults with COPD. This short low-pitched sound is often mistaken for whimpering and suggests severe hypoxia.

2. **(B)** Respiratory acidosis is caused by excess carbon dioxide retention.

3. **(C)** The absence of carbon dioxide likely indicates that the endotracheal tube has been placed in the esophagus. Verifying correct endotracheal tube placement is absolutely essential. $ETCO_2$ is only one method to assist in verification.

4. **(D)** The endotracheal tube is likely placed in the esophagus. Your next action is to remove the endotracheal tube and provide several ventilations with supplemental oxygen prior to attempting another intubation.

5. **(D)** All of the above. Vecuronium is a common nondepolarizing neuromuscular blocker. Succinylcholine is a common depolarizing neuromuscular blocker. Lidocaine is commonly used in RSI to prevent dysrhythmias associated with stimulation of the glottis associated with intubation. Atropine is often administered to decrease the incidence of bradycardia associated with the administration of succinylcholine.

6. **(D)** Of the choices listed, insertion of an oropharyngeal airway and ventilating with a bag-valve device is the best answer. **(A)** is incorrect because the oxygen flow setting is too low, it should be at least 15 LPM. **(B)** is incorrect because it utilizes a nonrebreather mask to assist ventilations. Nonrebreathers are not designed for or capable of assisting ventilations. **(C)** is incorrect because an apneic patient cannot be nasotracheally intubated.

7. **(D)** None of the above are correct. **(A)** is incorrect because both devices require assessment for accurate placement. With the PTL you begin ventilation through a short tube (the one without the stylet); with the Combitube, you begin ventilation through a longer blue tube. If chest rise and presence of breath sounds are not observed, you must switch immediately to the other ventilation port and reassess. **(B)** is incorrect because both are inserted in the neutral position and no manipulation of the head and neck is required for insertion. **(C)** is incorrect because both devices are inserted blindly.

8. **(B)** Adventitious breath sounds are considered abnormal sounds such as crackles and rhonchi.

9. **(C)** This is a simple anatomy and physiology question. The nose, nasal cavities, nasopharynx, oropharynx, laryngopharynx, larynx, and trachea correctly describe the flow of air.

10. **(D)** Breathing must be supported with a bag-valve device with supplemental high-flow oxygen. This patient's breathing is too slow and too shallow to receive enough oxygen for proper gas exchange to take place.

11. **(C)** The normal arterial pH range in the human body is: 7.35–7.45.

12. **(B)** This patient was most likely intubated in the right mainstem bronchus. Deflating the endotracheal tube cuff, withdrawing the tube slightly, reinflating the cuff, and reevaluating breath sounds is the proper procedure when a right mainstem bronchus intubation is suspected.

13. **(C)** Posterior pressure exerted on the cricoid cartilage (the Sellick maneuver) will effectively compress the esophagus, minimizing the potential for gastric distention. This maneuver will also reposition the vocal cords for clearer visualization of anatomic structures.

14. **(C)** This is a basic anatomy and physiology question. The area where the trachea divides into the right and left mainstem bronchi is known as the carina.

15. **(D)** Morphine is an opiate that can cause central nervous system depression. Administration may result in a decrease in the respiratory rate. Patients receiving morphine must be monitored closely for respiratory depression.

16. **(B)** The anatomical structure between the base of the tongue and the epiglottis into which the tip of the curved blade is placed during orotracheal intubation is the vallecula.

17. **(C)** Vesicular breath sounds are defined as normal sounds heard over most of the chest wall.

18. **(B)** Rate and depth of respiration are increased to eliminate excess CO_2 and therefore decreasing hydrogen ion concentrations. This is a normal compensatory mechanism of the body.

19. **(D)** Erythrocytes are defined as the blood component responsible for transporting oxygen from the lungs to the body tissues and transporting carbon dioxide from the tissues to the lungs.

20. **(A)** LMA insertion does not require laryngoscopy. **(B)** is incorrect because the LMA isolates the trachea, not the esophagus. **(C)** is a factual statement but is not an advantage of the LMA. Regurgitation and aspiration is the most significant complication associated with LMA use. **(D)** is incorrect. An intact gag reflex increases the likelihood of vomiting and aspiration.

21. **(B)** Hypoxic drive to breathe is common in patients with COPD or other degenerative respiratory disorders. Hypoxic drive is regulated by a low PaO_2 (partial pressure of oxygen). Delivering an increased concentration of oxygen may increase the PaO_2 and therefore eliminate the drive to breathe.

22. **(B)** When gastric distension interferes with ventilations, insertion of a naso/oral gastric tube into the stomach is indicated.

23. **(A)** This is a basic airway management question. The head-tilt/chin-lift maneuver is the simplest airway management technique to open the airway when no cervical spine trauma is suspected.

24. **(C)** The proper size oropharyngeal airway (OPA) is determined by measuring from the corner of the mouth to the tip of the earlobe at the angle of the jaw. It is essential that the OPA be sized appropriately because improper sizing can lead to airway obstruction.

25. **(C)** The normal value for PCO_2 is 35 to 45 mmHg. A high PCO_2 is considered respiratory acidosis. A low PCO_2 is considered respiratory alkalosis.

26. **(B)** The valve opening at the cardiac sphincter (opening into the stomach) is approximately 30 cm/H_2O. Not exceeding 30 cm/H_2O will reduce (not eliminate) the occurrence of gastric distension.

27. **(C)** Don't forget the basics! The head-tilt/chin-lift and jaw-thrust maneuver are both manual airway maneuvers that are very effective in initial management of the airway.

28. **(A)** CPAP/BiPAP has been proven to decrease the intubation rate in patients who previously required intubation. **(B)** is incorrect. Several contraindications exist for its use. **(C)** is incorrect. The patient must be breathing on his/her own to receive CPAP/BiPAP.

29. **(A)** The sniffing position is not required to perform digital intubation. The head can remain in a neutral position, therefore digital intubation may be helpful with suspected spinal cord injury. **(B)** is incorrect because the ET tube is inserted into the trachea using the index finger as a leverage point. A swollen tongue would make this difficult. **(C)** is incorrect. If the patient is breathing, digital intubation is contraindicated. **(D)** is incorrect. If airway obstruction is suspected, the obstruction needs to be removed or cricothyrotomy may need to be performed.

30. **(D)** The Esophageal Tracheal CombiTube is not indicated for pediatric patients due to its large diameter and the risk of perforation of the esophagus.

31. **(D)** All the conditions listed will result in a decreased $ETCO_2$ reading. Other causes include shock, bronchospasm, and incomplete airway obstruction (such as mucus plugging).

32. **(D)** Remember the basics! You must first open the airway and suction it before any other airway management.

33. **(C)** Endotracheal intubation is the only choice that is correct. **(A)** is incorrect because you do not ventilate through a nonrebreather mask. **(B)** is incorrect because the ventilation rate is too fast. **(D)** is incorrect because a patient must be breathing to receive oxygen through a nonrebreather mask.

34. **(B)** Succinylcholine should not be used in blunt trauma, burns, or crush injuries because these conditions can result in hyperkalemia. **(A)** is incorrect. Caution should be used if hypovolemia is present, but it is not contraindicated. **(C)** is incorrect. Succinylcholine is a depolarizing neuromuscular blocker. **(D)** is incorrect. Laryngeal edema is not a contraindication.

35. **(A)** CO_2 is a very potent vasodilator. When a patient is hyperventilated, CO_2 is removed and the vessels will become constricted. This vasoconstriction leads to decreased cerebral pressure by decreasing cerebral blood flow.

36. **(A)** This is a trauma victim and should be managed utilizing c-spine precautions. **(A)** is the only correct answer. Using any other option would potentiate a cervical spine injury.

37. **(D)** Clear lung sounds do not indicate the presence of a tension pneumothorax.

38. **(D)** In a tension pneumothorax, the patient is dealing with oxygenation problems and circulation problems. The tension pneumothorax creates an intrathoracic shift, impeding venous blood return to the heart.

39. **(A)** During needle decompression, the needle is inserted on top of the third rib to ensure that the vein, artery, and nerve bundle under each rib are not damaged. Each intercostal space contains a vein, artery, and nerve, which lie underneath each rib.

40. **(C)** In this scenario, suctioning is indicated. A patient with chronic bronchitis produces copious amounts of mucus, which is capable of plugging the larger airways of an ET tube. This would result in difficult ventilations. **(A)** is incorrect. Increasing the ventilation rate does not correct the problem. **(B)** is incorrect because breath sounds are equal. Gastric decompression **(D)** could be considered but not before suctioning; therefore **(D)** is not the best answer choice.

41. **(B)** Pulsus paradoxus is defined as a drop in systolic blood pressure of 10 mmHg or more, or the absence of a radial pulse during inspiration.

42. **(B)** A nasal cannula will deliver 40% of oxygen at a flow rate of 6 LPM in optimal conditions.

43. **(D)** A nonrebreather mask can deliver an oxygen concentration of 90–100% at a flow rate of 15 LPM.

44. **(D)** A bag-valve-mask device with a reservoir and an adequate oxygen source (at least 15 LPM) will deliver an oxygen concentration of 100%.

45. **(B)** The minimum size bag-valve mask device used for neonates, infants, and children should be 450 ml. Although it is likely that the bag-valve-mask will not deliver 450 ml of volume, it is important to have a device capable of delivering excessive volumes because, as the bag is compressed, there is dead space, from which air cannot be fully expelled.

46. **(B)** This patient needs oxygen by nonrebreather mask. He has an increased respiratory rate and PVCs on the monitor that may indicate hypoxia. A normal pulse oximeter of 97% is an excellent finding but oxygen should not be withheld based on this reading. Always remember to treat your patient and not the pulse oximeter.

47. **(B)** Prolonged suctioning has been found to cause hypoxia; therefore, suctioning should be limited to extraction only.

48. **(B)** The nasopharyngeal airway should be measured from the tip of the nose to the earlobe.

49. **(A)** When using a straight blade to intubate an adult patient, the tip of the blade should be placed directly on or under the epiglottis.

50. **(B)** When intubating an adult patient with a curved blade, the tip of the blade should be placed in the vallecula, at the base of the tongue.

51. **(D)** Auscultating individual lung fields is of great benefit because they help to confirm tube placement. Auscultation of the epigastrium is beneficial because it will help to verify improper tube placement or problems with the cuff seal of the tube.

52. **(A)** Cheyne-Stokes respiratory pattern is characterized by a gradually increasing rate and tidal volume followed by a gradual decrease with intermittent periods of apnea. This breathing pattern is usually seen in patients with brain injury or elderly patients with terminal illness.

53. **(B)** Biot's respiratory pattern is characterized by an irregular pattern, rate, and volume with intermittent periods of apnea. This pattern is seen in patients with increased intracranial pressure.

54. **(C)** Central neurogenic hyperventilation respiratory pattern is characterized by deep, rapid respirations. This breathing pattern is usually seen in a loss of normal regulation of ventilatory control.

55. **(D)** Bradypnea respiratory pattern is characterized by slow, shallow, irregular respirations. This breathing pattern can be associated with stroke or several other nervous system diseases.

56. **(D)** Hyperthermia (fever) should not affect the accuracy of a pulse oximeter reading. Other circumstances that can affect accuracy include exposure to nail polish or acrylic nails, dark pigmentation or bruising, high bilirubin concentration.

57. **(B)** Gastric distension usually occurs with bag-valve mask ventilations prior to intubation. A correctly placed endotracheal tube should not contribute to gastric distension.

58. **(D)** Current recommendations for confirmation of endotracheal tube placement should be evaluated immediately after insertion, each time the patient is moved, and by at least two methods.

59. **(C)** Stridor is defined as a high-pitched noise associated with upper airway constriction. This can be an indication of pending complete airway obstruction when associated with conditions such as anaphylactic shock.

Questions 60 to 65 are basic life support questions. If you miss any of these questions, it is essential to review basic CPR prior to taking your exam.

60. **(C)** looking, listening, and feeling airflow through the victim's nose or mouth.

61. **(B)** One breath every 5 seconds.

62. **(C)** On the lower half of the sternum, at the nipple line.

63. **(C)** 30 compressions to 2 ventilations.

64. **(A)** 100 times per minute.

65. **(A)** Once every 3 seconds (20 times per minute).

66. **(B)** A patient not being able to speak in full sentences due to breathing difficulty indicates that the patient does not have an adequate tidal volume. This assessment finding can be a significant warning sign of pending respiratory failure.

67. **(D)** Pursed-lip breathing technique helps maintain pressure within the airways (even during exhalation) to support bronchial walls that have been damaged as a result of disease.

68. **(C)** Cyanosis is correct because the question asks about significant decompensation. Decreased level of consciousness **(A)**, is an *early* indicator of decompensation. Proper care should be instituted to hopefully prevent the development of significant decompensation. This is an example of how test-taking skills come in handy. You must understand what the question is asking in order to choose the correct answer. **(B)** and **(D)** may or may not be present depending on the cause of the respiratory difficulty.

69. **(A)** Based on the history of the patient choking, a constant cough (from broncho spasm), and diminished breath sounds (obstruction) on the right should lead you to suspect aspiration of food.

70. **(C)** A suspected basilar skull fracture is a contraindication for nasotracheal intubation because the distal tip of the endotracheal tube could enter the cranial cavity through the fracture site.

71. **(C)** Blind nasotracheal intubation requires the patient to have spontaneous respirations because the endotracheal tube is inserted as the patient inhales.

72. **(B)** Suctioning should not exceed 5 seconds in an infant, 10 seconds in a child, and 15 seconds in an adult.

73. **(C)** There is no escaping the fact that the body becomes less efficient with age. Decreased chest wall compliance, loss of lung elasticity, air trapping, decreased diffusion of gases, and hypertrophy of the respiratory muscles can all contribute to a less effective respiratory system in a geriatric patient.

74. **(B)** This patient was most likely intubated in the right mainstem bronchus. Deflating the endotracheal tube cuff, withdrawing the tube slightly, reinflating the cuff, and reevaluating breath sounds is the proper procedure when a right mainstem bronchus intubation is suspected.

75. **(D)** Hyperthermia will not cause the pulse oximeter error.

76. **(A)** Field extubation is not common. If it must be performed, the patient must clearly be able to maintain and protect his or her own airway and have adequate spontaneous respirations.

77. **(C)** The endotracheal tube must be removed swiftly on a cough or expiration.

78. **(B)** A patient with a pulse oximeter reading of 86% with no significant past medical history of pulmonary disorders is considered hypoxic.

79. **(D)** Rhonchi are abnormal lung sounds heard on auscultation of airway that is obstructed by thick secretions.

80. **(C)** If the endotracheal tube has been placed in the esophagus, inflating the cuff on the endotracheal tube will hold the esophagus open and allow the bulb syringe to inflate. It is important to *not* inflate the endotracheal tube cuff prior to using any bulb syringe device.

Notes

Notes

Cardiology

 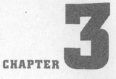

Cardiovascular disease is the leading cause of death in the United States. It also accounts for a large volume of EMS transports each year. It is essential for you to have a stable foundation of cardiovascular assessment, recognition, and treatment concepts.

All ECG rhythm strips used in this chapter are six-second strips.

Answer Sheet
CHAPTER 3—CARDIOLOGY

1 Ⓐ Ⓑ Ⓒ Ⓓ	33 Ⓐ Ⓑ Ⓒ Ⓓ	65 Ⓐ Ⓑ Ⓒ Ⓓ	97 Ⓐ Ⓑ Ⓒ Ⓓ
2 Ⓐ Ⓑ Ⓒ Ⓓ	34 Ⓐ Ⓑ Ⓒ Ⓓ	66 Ⓐ Ⓑ Ⓒ Ⓓ	98 Ⓐ Ⓑ Ⓒ Ⓓ
3 Ⓐ Ⓑ Ⓒ Ⓓ	35 Ⓐ Ⓑ Ⓒ Ⓓ	67 Ⓐ Ⓑ Ⓒ Ⓓ	99 Ⓐ Ⓑ Ⓒ Ⓓ
4 Ⓐ Ⓑ Ⓒ Ⓓ	36 Ⓐ Ⓑ Ⓒ Ⓓ	68 Ⓐ Ⓑ Ⓒ Ⓓ	100 Ⓐ Ⓑ Ⓒ Ⓓ
5 Ⓐ Ⓑ Ⓒ Ⓓ	37 Ⓐ Ⓑ Ⓒ Ⓓ	69 Ⓐ Ⓑ Ⓒ Ⓓ	101 Ⓐ Ⓑ Ⓒ Ⓓ
6 Ⓐ Ⓑ Ⓒ Ⓓ	38 Ⓐ Ⓑ Ⓒ Ⓓ	70 Ⓐ Ⓑ Ⓒ Ⓓ	102 Ⓐ Ⓑ Ⓒ Ⓓ
7 Ⓐ Ⓑ Ⓒ Ⓓ	39 Ⓐ Ⓑ Ⓒ Ⓓ	71 Ⓐ Ⓑ Ⓒ Ⓓ	103 Ⓐ Ⓑ Ⓒ Ⓓ
8 Ⓐ Ⓑ Ⓒ Ⓓ	40 Ⓐ Ⓑ Ⓒ Ⓓ	72 Ⓐ Ⓑ Ⓒ Ⓓ	104 Ⓐ Ⓑ Ⓒ Ⓓ
9 Ⓐ Ⓑ Ⓒ Ⓓ	41 Ⓐ Ⓑ Ⓒ Ⓓ	73 Ⓐ Ⓑ Ⓒ Ⓓ	105 Ⓐ Ⓑ Ⓒ Ⓓ
10 Ⓐ Ⓑ Ⓒ Ⓓ	42 Ⓐ Ⓑ Ⓒ Ⓓ	74 Ⓐ Ⓑ Ⓒ Ⓓ	106 Ⓐ Ⓑ Ⓒ Ⓓ
11 Ⓐ Ⓑ Ⓒ Ⓓ	43 Ⓐ Ⓑ Ⓒ Ⓓ	75 Ⓐ Ⓑ Ⓒ Ⓓ	107 Ⓐ Ⓑ Ⓒ Ⓓ
12 Ⓐ Ⓑ Ⓒ Ⓓ	44 Ⓐ Ⓑ Ⓒ Ⓓ	76 Ⓐ Ⓑ Ⓒ Ⓓ	108 Ⓐ Ⓑ Ⓒ Ⓓ
13 Ⓐ Ⓑ Ⓒ Ⓓ	45 Ⓐ Ⓑ Ⓒ Ⓓ	77 Ⓐ Ⓑ Ⓒ Ⓓ	109 Ⓐ Ⓑ Ⓒ Ⓓ
14 Ⓐ Ⓑ Ⓒ Ⓓ	46 Ⓐ Ⓑ Ⓒ Ⓓ	78 Ⓐ Ⓑ Ⓒ Ⓓ	110 Ⓐ Ⓑ Ⓒ Ⓓ
15 Ⓐ Ⓑ Ⓒ Ⓓ	47 Ⓐ Ⓑ Ⓒ Ⓓ	79 Ⓐ Ⓑ Ⓒ Ⓓ	111 Ⓐ Ⓑ Ⓒ Ⓓ
16 Ⓐ Ⓑ Ⓒ Ⓓ	48 Ⓐ Ⓑ Ⓒ Ⓓ	80 Ⓐ Ⓑ Ⓒ Ⓓ	112 Ⓐ Ⓑ Ⓒ Ⓓ
17 Ⓐ Ⓑ Ⓒ Ⓓ	49 Ⓐ Ⓑ Ⓒ Ⓓ	81 Ⓐ Ⓑ Ⓒ Ⓓ	113 Ⓐ Ⓑ Ⓒ Ⓓ
18 Ⓐ Ⓑ Ⓒ Ⓓ	50 Ⓐ Ⓑ Ⓒ Ⓓ	82 Ⓐ Ⓑ Ⓒ Ⓓ	114 Ⓐ Ⓑ Ⓒ Ⓓ
19 Ⓐ Ⓑ Ⓒ Ⓓ	51 Ⓐ Ⓑ Ⓒ Ⓓ	83 Ⓐ Ⓑ Ⓒ Ⓓ	115 Ⓐ Ⓑ Ⓒ Ⓓ
20 Ⓐ Ⓑ Ⓒ Ⓓ	52 Ⓐ Ⓑ Ⓒ Ⓓ	84 Ⓐ Ⓑ Ⓒ Ⓓ	116 Ⓐ Ⓑ Ⓒ Ⓓ
21 Ⓐ Ⓑ Ⓒ Ⓓ	53 Ⓐ Ⓑ Ⓒ Ⓓ	85 Ⓐ Ⓑ Ⓒ Ⓓ	117 Ⓐ Ⓑ Ⓒ Ⓓ
22 Ⓐ Ⓑ Ⓒ Ⓓ	54 Ⓐ Ⓑ Ⓒ Ⓓ	86 Ⓐ Ⓑ Ⓒ Ⓓ	118 Ⓐ Ⓑ Ⓒ Ⓓ
23 Ⓐ Ⓑ Ⓒ Ⓓ	55 Ⓐ Ⓑ Ⓒ Ⓓ	87 Ⓐ Ⓑ Ⓒ Ⓓ	119 Ⓐ Ⓑ Ⓒ Ⓓ
24 Ⓐ Ⓑ Ⓒ Ⓓ	56 Ⓐ Ⓑ Ⓒ Ⓓ	88 Ⓐ Ⓑ Ⓒ Ⓓ	120 Ⓐ Ⓑ Ⓒ Ⓓ
25 Ⓐ Ⓑ Ⓒ Ⓓ	57 Ⓐ Ⓑ Ⓒ Ⓓ	89 Ⓐ Ⓑ Ⓒ Ⓓ	121 Ⓐ Ⓑ Ⓒ Ⓓ
26 Ⓐ Ⓑ Ⓒ Ⓓ	58 Ⓐ Ⓑ Ⓒ Ⓓ	90 Ⓐ Ⓑ Ⓒ Ⓓ	122 Ⓐ Ⓑ Ⓒ Ⓓ
27 Ⓐ Ⓑ Ⓒ Ⓓ	59 Ⓐ Ⓑ Ⓒ Ⓓ	91 Ⓐ Ⓑ Ⓒ Ⓓ	123 Ⓐ Ⓑ Ⓒ Ⓓ
28 Ⓐ Ⓑ Ⓒ Ⓓ	60 Ⓐ Ⓑ Ⓒ Ⓓ	92 Ⓐ Ⓑ Ⓒ Ⓓ	124 Ⓐ Ⓑ Ⓒ Ⓓ
29 Ⓐ Ⓑ Ⓒ Ⓓ	61 Ⓐ Ⓑ Ⓒ Ⓓ	93 Ⓐ Ⓑ Ⓒ Ⓓ	125 Ⓐ Ⓑ Ⓒ Ⓓ
30 Ⓐ Ⓑ Ⓒ Ⓓ	62 Ⓐ Ⓑ Ⓒ Ⓓ	94 Ⓐ Ⓑ Ⓒ Ⓓ	
31 Ⓐ Ⓑ Ⓒ Ⓓ	63 Ⓐ Ⓑ Ⓒ Ⓓ	95 Ⓐ Ⓑ Ⓒ Ⓓ	
32 Ⓐ Ⓑ Ⓒ Ⓓ	64 Ⓐ Ⓑ Ⓒ Ⓓ	96 Ⓐ Ⓑ Ⓒ Ⓓ	

1. Which term best describes the following definition? Disease of arterial vessels marked by thickening, hardening, and loss of elasticity in the arterial walls.
   (A) Atherosclerosis
   (B) Arterionecrosis
   (C) Arteriosclerosis
   (D) Angina

2. The point of maximal impulse (PMI) can usually be felt on the
   (A) medial aspect of the chest, just below the fourth intercostal space.
   (B) left anterior chest, in the midclavicular line, at the fifth intercostal space.
   (C) left lateral chest, in the midaxillary line, at the fourth intercostal space.
   (D) left anterior chest, in the midaxillary line, at the fifth intercostal space.

3. The volume of blood ejected from the left ventricle into the arterial system each minute is
   (A) preload.
   (B) cardiac output.
   (C) afterload.
   (D) stroke volume.

4. Administering a drug with a positive chronotropic effect will have a direct effect on the
   (A) ejection fraction.
   (B) blood pressure.
   (C) cardiac output.
   (D) heart rate.

5. The resistance against which the heart must pump is
   (A) afterload.
   (B) blood pressure.
   (C) preload.
   (D) cardiac output.

6. The amount of blood ejected from the heart in one cardiac contraction is
   (A) cardiac output.
   (B) stroke volume.
   (C) preload.
   (D) afterload.

7. Hypocalcemia and hypomagnesemia would MOST likely result in
   (A) decreased cardiac conduction.
   (B) increased myocardial irritability.
   (C) decreased cardiac contractility.
   (D) decreased myocardial automaticity.

8. The protective sac surrounding the heart is the
   (A) myocardium.
   (B) septum.
   (C) endocardium.
   (D) pericardium.

9. Which of the following medications has beta-2-specific properties?
   (A) Dopamine
   (B) Levophed
   (C) Proventil
   (D) Epinephrine

10. When a 12-lead ECG is obtained for patients with chest pain, it is important to consider that
    (A) it may take hours for changes to appear on the ECG.
    (B) an unremarkable 12-lead ECG rules out an acute MI.
    (C) the 12-lead alone should be used to guide your treatment.
    (D) the ECG's analysis of the rhythm is more accurate than yours.

11. When assessing a 12-lead ECG to confirm ischemia or injury to the heart, you must see evidence in ____ or more contiguous leads.
    (A) two
    (B) three
    (C) four
    (D) five

12. Which of the following statements is MOST correct?
    (A) Lead I is contiguous with lead II.
    (B) Lead II is contiguous with leads V_6 and aVL.
    (C) Lead V_6 is contiguous with leads V_4 and V_5.
    (D) Lead V_6 is contiguous with lead V_5 and lead I.

13. When assessing a 12-lead ECG, acute infarction to the inferior wall of the myocardium would present as
    (A) pathologic Q waves in leads V_4 and V_5.
    (B) ST segment elevation in leads II, III, and aVF.
    (C) T-wave inversion in leads V_1 through V_4.
    (D) ST segment depression in leads II and III.

14. When assessing a 12-lead ECG, ischemia to the anterior wall of the myocardium would present as
    (A) T-wave inversion in leads V_3 and V_4.
    (B) ST segment depression in leads I and aVL.
    (C) T-wave inversion in leads II, III, and aVF.
    (D) ST segment elevation in leads V_3 and V_4.

15. When assessing a 12-lead ECG, a pathologic Q wave:
    (A) generally indicates that an acute MI has occurred within the past hour.
    (B) is deeper than one half of the height of the R wave and indicates injury.
    (C) is wider than 0.04 second and is seen in two or more contiguous leads.
    (D) can be substantiated only by comparing two previous 12-lead ECGs.

16. When assessing a 12-lead ECG, leads V_1 to V_3 allow you to view the
    _____ wall of the left ventricle.
    (A) anterolateral
    (B) lateral
    (C) septal
    (D) anteroseptal

17. In a patient experiencing chest pain, the presence of jugular venous distention while sitting at a 45° angle
    (A) is not clinically significant.
    (B) requires CPAP for treatment.
    (C) suggests left side heart failure.
    (D) indicates right heart compromise.

18. Which of the following medications would be the MOST acceptable alternative to morphine for analgesia in patients with an acute coronary syndrome?
    (A) Versed
    (B) Fentanyl
    (C) Diazepam
    (D) Narcan

19. In Lead II, placement of the positive lead is located on the
    (A) left arm.
    (B) right shoulder.
    (C) right leg.
    (D) left leg.

20. In Lead III placement, the positive lead is located on the
    (A) left arm.
    (B) right shoulder.
    (C) right leg.
    (D) left leg.

21. _____ seconds are measured in each small square on ECG graph paper.
    (A) 0.01
    (B) 0.4
    (C) 0.04
    (D) 0.20

22. _____ seconds are measured in each large box on ECG graph paper.
    (A) 0.01
    (B) 0.4
    (C) 0.04
    (D) 0.20

23. A normal PR interval is _____ to _____ seconds.
    (A) 0.04–0.10
    (B) 0.08–0.10
    (C) 0.10–0.20
    (D) 0.12–0.20

24. The duration of a normal QRS complex is _____ seconds.
    (A) 0.12–0.20
    (B) 0.10–0.20
    (C) 0.04–0.10
    (D) 0.08–0.12

25. The intrinsic firing rate for a ventricular pacemaker is _____ beats per minute.
    (A) 20 to 40
    (B) 40 to 60
    (C) 60 to 100
    (D) 100 to 150

26. The time elapsing between the beginning of the P wave and the beginning of the QRS complex on the electrocardiogram is the
    (A) QRS complex.
    (B) first-degree heart block.
    (C) QT interval.
    (D) PR interval.

27. The return of a cardiac muscle cell to its resting state is called
    (A) synapse.
    (B) depolarization.
    (C) repolarization.
    (D) automaticity.

28. In a normal heart, the pacemaker cell is
    (A) the atrioventricular node.
    (B) Purkinje fibers.
    (C) the sinoatrial node.
    (D) the internodal pathways.

29. The SA node is located
    (A) high in the right atrium.
    (B) high in the left atrium.
    (C) in the septum.
    (D) high in the left ventricle.

30. Which of the following is not part of the heart's electrical conduction system that contains pacemaking capabilities?
    (A) Bundle of His
    (B) Purkinje system
    (C) SA node
    (D) AV node

31. The intrinsic firing rate of the AV node is
    (A) 20–40 beats per minute.
    (B) 40–60 beats per minute.
    (C) 40–80 beats per minute.
    (D) 60–100 beats per minute.

32. On an ECG tracing, the P wave indicates
    (A) depolarization of the atria.
    (B) repolarization of the atria.
    (C) depolarization of the ventricles.
    (D) repolarization of the ventricles.

33. On an ECG tracing, the QRS complex indicates
    (A) depolarization of the atria.
    (B) repolarization of the atria.
    (C) depolarization of the ventricles.
    (D) repolarization of the ventricles.

34. On an ECG tracing, the T wave indicates
    (A) depolarization of the atria.
    (B) repolarization of the atria.
    (C) depolarization of the ventricles.
    (D) repolarization of the ventricles.

35. The time for an electrical impulse to be transmitted from the atria to the ventricles is the
    (A) PR interval.
    (B) T wave.
    (C) QRS complex.
    (D) J point.

36. The period of the cardiac cycle when stimulation will not produce depolarization is the
    (A) refractory period.
    (B) decompensation period.
    (C) absolute refractory period.
    (D) relative refractory period.

37. The period of the cardiac cycle when stimulation may produce depolarization is the
    (A) refractory period.
    (B) decompensation period.
    (C) absolute refractory period.
    (D) relative refractory period.

38. Stimulation of the vagus nerve may result in
    (A) vasodilatation.
    (B) an increase in heart rate.
    (C) a decrease in heart rate.
    (D) an increase in cardiac output.

39. A rapid heart rate or irregular heartbeat may cause the patient to experience a sensation commonly known as
    (A) palpitations.
    (B) dysrhythmia.
    (C) fainting.
    (D) anxiety.

40. Cardiogenic shock can result in all of the following except
    (A) dysrhythmias.
    (B) hypertension.
    (C) respiratory failure.
    (D) an elevated heart rate.

41. The presence of pulmonary congestion indicated by abnormal lung sounds such as crackles (rales) in a patient complaining of chest pain may indicate
    (A) hypotension.
    (B) increased vagal tone.
    (C) increased stroke volume.
    (D) left ventricular failure.

42. Management of chest pain of a suspected cardiac nature includes
    (A) establishing an IV and providing a 200 cc fluid bolus.
    (B) administering Lasix 100 mg slow IV.
    (C) administering 2 liters oxygen by nasal cannula.
    (D) administering nitroglycerin gr1/150 sublingual.

43. Initial management of left ventricular failure in the prehospital setting may include
    (A) application of CPAP.
    (B) increasing venous return to the heart.
    (C) administering IV furosemide and morphine.
    (D) administering 3 liters oxygen by nasal cannula.

44. Management of cardiogenic shock may include
    (A) administration of morphine.
    (B) administration of IV dopamine.
    (C) administration of nitroglycerin gr1/150 sublingual.
    (D) establishing an IV 500 cc/hr.

45. Initial treatment for cardiac arrest due to ventricular fibrillation requires
    (A) one monophasic shock of 200 joules.
    (B) one biphasic shock of 120 joules.
    (C) administration of lidocaine.
    (D) administration of epinephrine.

46. Your patient is complaining of back and flank pain described as a tearing sensation. Inspection of the abdomen reveals a pulsatile mass. Treatment includes
    (A) palpation of the mass.
    (B) gentle handling and rapid transport.
    (C) administration of Lasix 40 mg IV.
    (D) administering lidocaine 100 mg IV.

47. Procainamide administration should be discontinued if which of the following occurs?
    (A) Hypotension
    (B) Widening of the QRS complex
    (C) Maximum dose infused
    (D) All of the above

48. Which of the following medications is not indicated in the treatment of ventricular fibrillation?
    (A) Epinephrine
    (B) Adenosine
    (C) Lidocaine
    (D) Vasopressin

49. Which of the following may require synchronized cardioversion?
    (A) Pulseless ventricular tachycardia
    (B) Pulseless electrical activity
    (C) Ventricular fibrillation
    (D) PSVT

50. Your patient in ventricular tachycardia is lethargic, diaphoretic, and pale and has vomited once. His vital signs are: BP 54/P, pulse 184, respirations 14. Describe your management of this patient.
    (A) 200 cc fluid bolus, nitroglycerin gr1/150 sublingual, lidocaine.
    (B) ABCs, high-flow oxygen, cardioversion.
    (C) ABCs, high-flow oxygen, IV, Adenocard 6 mg IV.
    (D) Intubation, IV, dopamine infusion.

51. You respond to a 76-year-old man with syncope. He is sitting upright in the bathroom when you arrive. He stated that he was having a bowel movement when he blacked out. Based on the information provided, you suspect the cause of the patient's syncope is
    (A) digitalis toxicity.
    (B) an atrial dysrhythmia.
    (C) vasovagal episode.
    (D) underlying myocardial ischemia.

52. You respond to a possible drowning call. On arrival, you find bystander CPR in progress on a male patient in his thirties. Your first action should be
    (A) to take over CPR from the bystanders.
    (B) immediate defibrillation.
    (C) to stop bystander CPR to assess ABCs.
    (D) to open the airway and suction if necessary.

53. All of the following are treatable causes of pulseless electrical activity except
    (A) hypothermia, hypovolemia, cardiac tamponade, acidosis.
    (B) hypovolemia, tension pneumothorax, hyperthermia, hyperkalemia.
    (C) acidosis, coronary thrombosis, pulmonary embolism.
    (D) tension pneumothorax, hyperkalemia, coronary thrombosis.

54. You respond to a 20-year-old female complaining of dizziness and weakness. She is slow to respond to your questions but admits to taking several diet pills a day in an effort to quickly lose weight. Vitals are blood pressure 98/54, pulse 184, respirations 32; the skin is pale and moist. ECG shows the following rhythm:

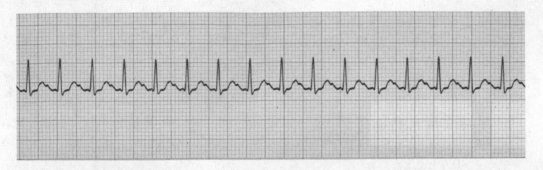

Immediate treatment should include
(A) reassuring the patient that when the medication wears off the symptoms will go away.
(B) IV, oxygen, continuing to monitor the patient, and transport.
(C) IV, oxygen, adenocard 6 mg rapid IV push.
(D) immediate cardioversion with 100 joules.

Questions 55 and 56 are based on the following scenario:

A 68-year-old woman is complaining of chest pain and shortness of breath. Her blood pressure is 110/64, pulse 60, respirations 32. ECG shows sinus bradycardia with a PR interval of 0.24. Lung sounds reveal crackles in the posterior bases.

55. Management should include
(A) nitroglycerin gr1/150 mg SL.
(B) a 200 cc fluid bolus.
(C) Atropine 0.5 mg to 1.0 mg IVP.
(D) preparation for immediate transcutaneous pacing.

56. The BP is now 88/50, pulse 46, respirations 40. Lung sounds reveal increased pulmonary congestion. Continued management should include
(A) Atropine 0.5 mg to 1 mg.
(B) administering a 200 cc fluid bolus.
(C) administering Lasix 80 mg IVP.
(D) immediate transcutaneous pacing.

57. A patient is experiencing severe chest pain, shortness of breath and becomes unconscious. BP is 72/40 and the ECG shows the following rhythm:

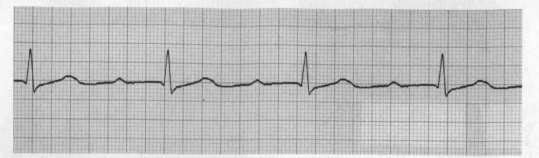

Treatment includes
(A) Atropine 0.5 mg IVP every five minutes to a maximum dose of 0.4 mg/kg.
(B) Dopamine infusion titrated to a systolic blood pressure >90 mmHg systolic.
(C) immediate transcutaneous pacing.
(D) 200 cc fluid bolus and rechecking vital signs.

Questions 58 and 59 are based on the following scenario:

A patient weighing 220 pounds presents in this rhythm:

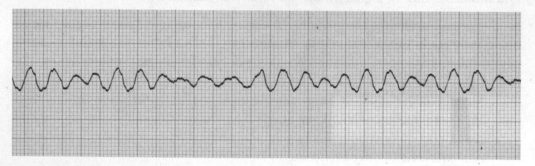

58. Management should include:
(A) amiodarone 300 mg IV.
(B) lidocaine 180 mg IV.
(C) procainamide 4 mg/min IV.
(D) magnesium 1 mg IV.

59. Further management for the rhythm includes:
    (A) amiodarone 150 mg IV.
    (B) vasopressin 20 mg IV.
    (C) procainamide 4 mg/min up to a total of 17 mg/kg IV.
    (D) magnesium 1 gram IV.

60. How often should you provide rescue breaths for a child who is apneic?
    (A) 12 to 20 breaths per minute
    (B) one breath every 5–6 seconds
    (C) after each pulse check
    (D) Once every 10 seconds

61. What is the proper rate of chest compressions to ventilations while performing two-person CPR on an adult with an advanced airway in place?
    (A) 30 compressions to 2 ventilations
    (B) 15 compressions to 1 ventilation
    (C) 15 compressions to 2 ventilations
    (D) 5 compressions to 2 ventilations

62. Calcium chloride is indicated for a dialysis patient in
    (A) cardiac arrest with refractory v fib.
    (B) symptomatic bradycardia.
    (C) cardiac arrest with known or suspected hyperkalemia.
    (D) cardiac arrest with asystole.

63. The recommended dose of vasopression in ventricular fibrillation is
    (A) 40 mg IV repeated once in 10 minutes.
    (B) 20 mg IV one time only.
    (C) 40 mg IV one time only.
    (D) 40 units IV one time only.

64. The maximum amount of procainamide you should administer to a 196-pound patient is
    (A) 1,462 mcg.
    (B) 1,500 mg.
    (C) 1,514 mg.
    (D) 1,615 mg.

65. The initial dose of adenosine that should be administered is
    (A) 6 mg rapid IV push, repeated in 5 minutes if necessary.
    (B) 6 mg IV push, repeated in 10 minutes.
    (C) 6 mg rapid IV push followed by a 20 cc fluid bolus.
    (D) 12 mg IV push.

66. The recommended dose of aspirin for a patient experiencing chest pain is
    (A) 325 mg.
    (B) 160–325 mg.
    (C) 81 mg.
    (D) 650 mg.

67. Mixing 2 grams of lidocaine in 500 cc of solution will provide a mixture of
    (A) 1 mg/ml.
    (B) 2 mg/ml.
    (C) 3 mg/ml.
    (D) 4 mg/ml.

68. To administer 2 mg/min of lidocaine using the mixture of 2 grams in 500 cc and 60 gtt/ml tubing, you will administer how many drops a minute?
    (A) 15
    (B) 30
    (C) 45
    (D) 60

69. You respond to a shopping mall for a possible cardiac arrest. When you arrive, you find a male patient in his seventies in cardiac arrest. The mall security officers have an AED attached. The AED is in the process of delivering a shock. Your first response should be to
    (A) establish unresponsiveness.
    (B) open the airway and provide ventilations.
    (C) remove the AED and apply your own monitor.
    (D) allow the AED to deliver the initial shock.

70. A dissecting aortic aneurysm may produce which signs/symptoms?
    (A) A ripping or tearing pain sensation
    (B) Pain in the abdomen
    (C) The same blood pressure in each arm
    (D) Respiratory distress

71. Vasopressin is indicated for management of
    (A) any circumstance in which epinephrine 1:10,000 may be used.
    (B) ventricular fibrillation.
    (C) PEA.
    (D) ventricular tachycardia with a pulse.

72. A 78-year-old male is alert and oriented to person, place, and time and complains of chest pain and difficulty breathing. You attach him to the ECG and notice a rhythm of 42 with corresponding pulse, a P-R interval of 0.20, and normal R-R intervals. Vitals are BP 76/42, respirations 42. The patient also states that he feels nauseated and dizzy. Treatment for this patient should include
    (A) atropine 0.5 mg.
    (B) oxygen 3 LPM nasal cannula.
    (C) immediate transvenous pacing.
    (D) Isuprel 2–10 mcg/min.

73. You encounter a patient with a P-R interval of 0.16, a QRS duration of 0.08, and a regular R-R interval. This patient is in
    (A) atrial fibrillation.
    (B) sinus rhythm with first-degree heart block.
    (C) sinus rhythm.
    (D) supraventricular tachycardia.

74. A 14-year-old female is crying and hysterical after breaking up with her boyfriend. She had a syncopal episode prior to EMS arrival. Vitals are BP 110/68, pulse 130, and respirations 36. You place her on the cardiac monitor and interpret the following rhythm as

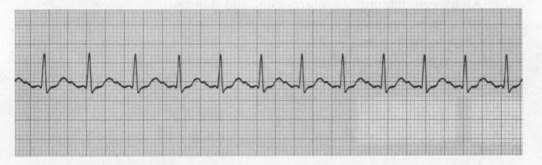

    (A) sinus arrest.
    (B) sinus bradycardia.
    (C) sinus dysrhythmia.
    (D) sinus tachycardia.

Question 75 and 76 are based on the following scenario:

A 62-year-old male fainted while working in the yard. His current vitals are BP 108/64, pulse 102 and irregular, and respirations 24. The ECG shows the following rhythm

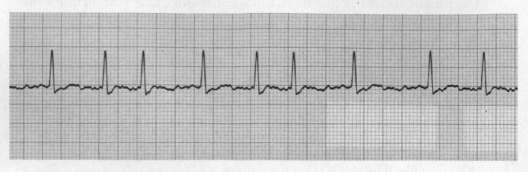

75. You interpret his ECG rhythm as
    (A) second-degree heart block.
    (B) sinus rhythm.
    (C) atrial fibrillation.
    (D) sinus bradycardia.

76. The patient complains of feeling that he is going to black out again. Vitals are unchanged. Treatment for the patient should include
    (A) oxygen, monitor, IV, observation, and transport.
    (B) oxygen, monitor, IV, Atropine.
    (C) oxygen, monitor, IV, Adenocard.
    (D) oxygen, monitor, IV, synchronized cardioversion.

Questions 77 and 78 are based on the following scenario:

EMS is called to the scene of a 72-year-old male with a history of cardiac disease. He is unconscious and unresponsive. BP is not obtainable, pulse 140 and weak, respirations 6. After placing him on the monitor, you note the following rhythm:

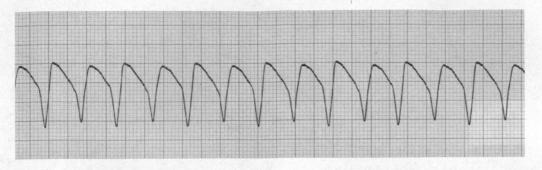

77. You interpret the rhythm as
    (A) supraventricular tachycardia.
    (B) ventricular tachycardia.
    (C) atrial fibrillation with a rapid ventricular response.
    (D) ventricular fibrillation.

78. Initial treatment of the patient should include
    (A) synchronized cardioversion.
    (B) defibrillation.
    (C) transcutaneous pacing.
    (D) Adenocard 6 mg IVP.

---

79. A healthy female is being transported for preterm labor contractions. Per protocol, she is lying slightly tilted on her left side, is on oxygen via nonrebreather mask, and an IV is established at KVO. You place her on the monitor and notice the following rhythm.

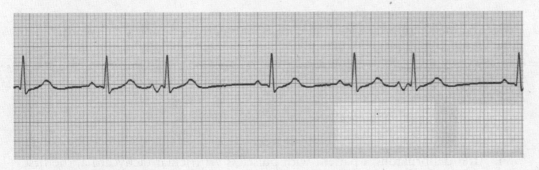

The rhythm is
(A) sinus rhythm with PACs.
(B) sinus rhythm with PJCs.
(C) sinus dysrhythmia.
(D) sinus rhythm with PVCs.

80. A 33-year-old man has just finished playing basketball. He is complaining of chest discomfort. Physical exam shows a rapid pulse, BP 128/64, respirations 30. ECG monitor shows the following rhythm:

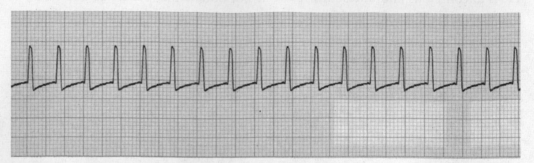

Treatment includes
(A) Adenocard 6 mg IV.
(B) cardioversion 100 joules.
(C) continuing to assess and monitor the patient.
(D) defibrillation.

81. All of the following are appropriate end points for procainamide administration except
(A) 17 mcg/kg administered.
(B) hypotension.
(C) widening of the QRS complex greater than 50%.
(D) the dysrhythmia is suppressed.

82. A patient experiencing a hypertensive crisis should receive the following medication:
(A) nitroglycerin.
(B) Procardia.
(C) aspirin.
(D) oxygen.

83. The medication treatment of choice for a narrow complex tachycardia in an unstable patient is
(A) Adenocard.
(B) lidocaine.
(C) cardioversion.
(D) Versed.

84. After defibrillating a patient with pulseless ventricular tachycardia, the first medication he or she should receive is
(A) epinephrine or vasopressin.
(B) lidocaine or amiodarone.
(C) epinephrine or lidocaine.
(D) vasopressin or amiodarone.

85. Vasopressin is useful in the management of
    (A) complete heart block.
    (B) PSVT.
    (C) ventricular fibrillation.
    (D) torsades v tach.

86. The recommended dose of vasopressin in v fib or pulseless v tach is
    (A) 17 mg/min IV infusion.
    (B) 2–4 mg/min IV infusion.
    (C) 40 units IV repeated once in 5 minutes.
    (D) 40 units IV in a single dose.

87. All of the following medications can be administered via endotracheal route except
    (A) lidocaine, atropine.
    (B) epinephrine, amiodarone.
    (C) oxygen, epinephrine.
    (D) Narcan, lidocaine.

88. A second dose of amiodarone is necessary for a patient in v fib. The dose to be administered is
    (A) 300 mg IV.
    (B) 150 mg IV.
    (C) 100 mg IV.
    (D) 40 units IV.

89. You arrive on scene of a 35-year-old male who is in distress. He is grabbing his throat with both hands. What should you do first?
    (A) Get behind him and perform the Heimlich maneuver.
    (B) Give five back blows.
    (C) Ask, "Are you choking?" and look for a response.
    (D) Alternate back blows with abdominal thrusts.

90. Acute coronary syndrome is defined as
    (A) a sudden ischemic disorder of the heart.
    (B) a myocardial infarction.
    (C) congestive heart failure.
    (D) triple vessel disease.

91. All of the following are considered anginal equivalents except
    (A) diaphoresis, syncope, dizziness.
    (B) dyspnea, palpitations, syncope.
    (C) hypoglycemia, chest pain, dyspnea.
    (D) fatigue, dizziness, palpitations.

92. Which signs/symptoms are considered atypical presentation of myocardial ischemia?
    (A) Lower extremity pain, shoulder pain, abdominal pain
    (B) Epigastric pain, reproducible pain, sharp or knifelike pain
    (C) Nausea, dizziness, palpitations
    (D) All of the above

93. Nitroglycerin has all of the following properties except
    (A) it prevents vasospasm.
    (B) it is a vasodilator.
    (C) it decreases afterload.
    (D) it decreases preload.

Questions 94 and 95 are based on the following scenario:

You respond to a patient with shortness of breath. The patient said he was awakened from his sleep with shortness of breath. Assessment reveals vitals: BP of 188/94, pulse 116, respiration 36, and a pulse oximeter reading of 88%. Lung sound assessment reveals crackles in the posterior bases.

94. You suspect this patient to be suffering from
    (A) a myocardial infarction.
    (B) angina.
    (C) congestive heart failure.
    (D) a respiratory disorder.

95. As you continue your assessment on this patient, he becomes lethargic. BP is now 198/102, pulse 136, respirations 48, with increased pulmonary congestion. Treatment should include
    (A) preparation for intubation.
    (B) preparation for immediate transcutaneous pacing.
    (C) CPAP at 10 cm H_2O.
    (D) lidocaine 1.0 mg/kg IVP.

96. A patient is experiencing severe chest pain and dyspnea. He is nauseated and extremely diaphoretic, BP is 78/42, pulse is tachycardic, and respirations 36. The patient weighs 190 pounds. ECG shows the following rhythm:

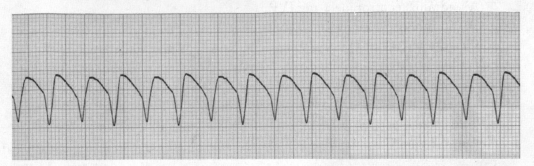

Initial treatment should include
(A) lidocaine 85 to 130 mg IVP.
(B) defibrillation.
(C) cardioversion.
(D) Adenocard 6 mg rapid IVP.

97. You are called for a patient with syncope. On arrival the patient is conscious. Vitals are BP 92/54, pulse 110, respirations 24. ECG shows the following rhythm:

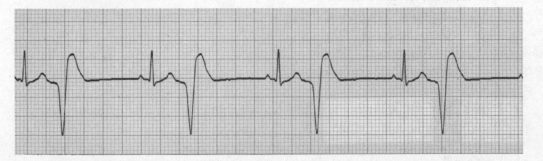

Which treatment is appropriate?
(A) Atropine 0.5 mg
(B) Immediate defibrillation
(C) Lidocaine 1.5 mg/kg
(D) Continued observation

98. You just administered atropine 0.5 mg for a patient with a symptomatic bradycardia and multifocal PVCs. Suddenly your patient becomes unconscious and goes into ventricular fibrillation. Your next action is to
(A) administer lidocaine 1.5 mg/kg.
(B) administer another 0.5 mg of atropine IVP.
(C) cardiovert.
(D) defibrillate.

99. You just delivered one shock to a patient in ventricular fibrillation. The monitor now shows asystole. You confirm in two leads. Your next action is to
    (A) administer atropine 1 mg IVP.
    (B) administer vasopressin 20 units IV.
    (C) administer fluid bolus 200 cc.
    (D) defibrillate.

100. A 22-year-old female has just finished jogging five miles. She is complaining of palpitations. Vitals are BP 112/68, pulse 148, respirations 32. She denies drug use. ECG shows the following rhythm:

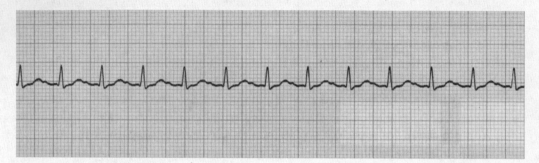

Treatment should include
    (A) adenosine 6 mg rapid IVP.
    (B) cardioversion at 100 joules.
    (C) vagal maneuver.
    (D) continued observation.

101. Which of the following rhythms require immediate transcutaneous pacing?
    (A) Junctional tachycardia
    (B) Sinus bradycardia with first-degree heart block
    (C) Supraventricular tachycardia
    (D) Third-degree AV block

102. When performing transcutaneous pacing, the paramedic should increase the _____delivered until mechanical capture is obtained.
    (A) joules
    (B) milliamps
    (C) rate
    (D) millivolts

103. You are called to a church where a 62-year-old male feels that his pacemaker is not functioning properly. He is conscious and alert but states that he is going to "pass out." You place him on your monitor and observe the following rhythm:

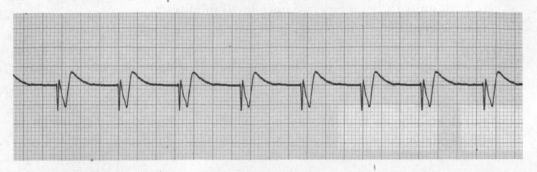

Treatment for this patient should include
(A) oxygen, IV, monitor, and continued observation.
(B) oxygen, IV, monitor, and lidocaine.
(C) oxygen, IV, monitor, nitroglycerin, and aspirin.
(D) oxygen, IV, monitor, cardioversion.

104. You arrive on scene of a patient who has had steadily worsening chest pain for four hours. He has taken 12 nitroglycerin with no relief. The best description of this type of chest pain is
(A) stable angina.
(B) unstable angina.
(C) Prinzmetal's angina.
(D) vasospastic angina.

105. You are evaluating a male patient with complaints of a "tearing sensation" epigastric pain. He tells you that the pain began two hours ago after eating lunch. He says he has never experienced any pain like this. He rates the pain as a 10, and states that it is radiating into his back and shoulder. Based on the information provided, you suspect the pain may be the result of
(A) a myocardial infarction.
(B) a hiatal hernia.
(C) an aortic aneurysm.
(D) gastric esophageal reflux disease.

106. The effect of dopamine administration at an infusion rate greater than 20 mcg/kg/minute includes
(A) arterial vasoconstriction only.
(B) venous vasoconstriction only.
(C) both arterial and venous peripheral vasoconstriction.
(D) improved renal blood flow.

107. The recommended dose of vasopressin in cardiac arrest due to pulseless VT or VF is:
    (A) 20 units IV bolus repeated once in 10 minutes.
    (B) a single IV bolus dose of 40 units.
    (C) 40 units IV bolus repeated once in 10 minutes.
    (D) 300 mg IV.

108. What is the initial dose for sodium bicarbonate administration?
    (A) 1 amp
    (B) 1 mEq/kg
    (C) 1 mcg/kg
    (D) 1 mg/kg

109. An unwanted side effect of dopamine administration includes
    (A) increased myocardial oxygen demand.
    (B) respiratory depression.
    (C) ventricular dysrhythmias.
    (D) dilation of renal vessels at high doses.

110. You have administered an initial dose of amiodarone for a patient in ventricular fibrillation. The repeat dose of this medication should be
    (A) 300 mg.
    (B) 150 mg.
    (C) 0.04 mg/kg.
    (D) 1 to 1.5 mg/kg.

111. Amiodarone
    (A) should be given by rapid IV infusion only.
    (B) may produce vasodilation and hypotension.
    (C) has a maximum dose of 17 mg/kg.
    (D) is indicated only in cardiac arrest.

112. Lidocaine may be lethal if administered to a patient with which of the following dysrhythmias?
    (A) Sinus rhythm with PACs
    (B) Second-degree AV block type I
    (C) Accelerated junctional rhythm
    (D) Second-degree AV block type II

113. A 68-year-old male suffered a syncopal episode while golfing. The cardiac monitor shows a sinus tachycardia at 142 beats/minute without ectopy. His blood pressure is presently 78/42. Despite a 200 cc fluid bolus the patient remains hypotensive. He has an altered mental status with cool and diaphoretic skin. Of the following, which is not likely to be considered for administration to this patient?
    (A) Dopamine
    (B) Nitroglycerin
    (C) A second fluid bolus
    (D) High-flow oxygen

114. Sodium bicarbonate administration may be useful for treating
    (A) beta-blocker overdoses and hypocalcemia.
    (B) preexisting acidosis and hypokalemia.
    (C) tricyclic antidepressant overdoses and hyperkalemia.
    (D) calcium channel blocker overdoses and hyperkalemia.

115. Before providing rescue breathing to an unresponsive victim, you must check for breathing. You do this by
    (A) opening the airway.
    (B) shaking and shouting to stimulate him or her to breathe.
    (C) looking, listening, and feeling the airflow through the victim's nose or mouth.
    (D) establishing unresponsiveness.

116. When performing CPR on an adult in cardiac arrest, it is important to
    (A) deliver at least 80 to 90 compressions per minute.
    (B) limit interruptions in chest compressions to 20 seconds.
    (C) deliver forceful ventilations between compressions.
    (D) allow the chest to fully recoil between compressions.

117. The proper compression-to-ventilation ratio for two-rescuer adult CPR when an oropharyngeal airway is in place is
    (A) 5:1.
    (B) 15:2.
    (C) 30:2.
    (D) asynchronous.

118. What is the ratio of chest compressions to ventilations when performing one-person CPR on an adult?
    (A) 5 compressions to 1 ventilation
    (B) 30 compressions to 1 ventilation
    (C) 30 compressions to 2 ventilations
    (D) 15 compressions to 2 ventilations

119. What is the speed you should use to perform chest compressions for an adult victim of cardiac arrest?
    (A) 60 times per minute
    (B) 80 times per minute
    (C) 100 times per minute
    (D) 120 times per minute

120. You arrive on the scene of a 56-year-old male patient who developed chest pain while mowing the lawn on a hot August day. He states the pain has subsided after a few minutes of rest. Your assessment shows that he is alert and oriented, BP 148/92, pulse 48, respirations of 20. His skin is warm and moist. He has no past medical history and takes no medications. You attach the monitor and observe the following rhythm:

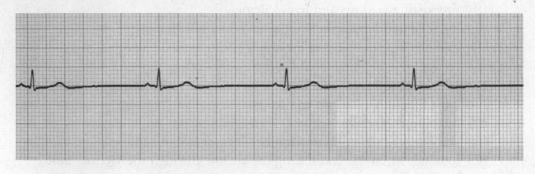

    Treatment should include
    (A) atropine 0.5 mg IVP.
    (B) Adenocard 5 mg IVP.
    (C) transport for evaluation.
    (D) No treatment is necessary.

121. A 70-year-old woman remains in asystole following 10 minutes of well-coordinated CPR, intubation, IV, and several rounds of medications. There are no obvious causes that would explain her cardiac arrest. At this point, it would be MOST appropriate to
    (A) attempt transcutaneous cardiac pacing.
    (B) defibrillate one time in case she is in v-fib.
    (C) transport while continuing CPR enroute.
    (D) consider ceasing resuscitative efforts.

122. Your chest pain patient suddenly becomes lethargic. BP is 82/40, pulse 36, respirations 10. You note the following rhythm on the monitor:

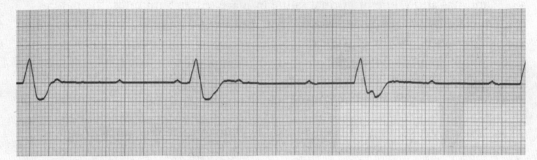

Treatment should include
(A) atropine 0.5 mg IV.
(B) Adenocard 5 mg IV.
(C) stopping nitroglycerin administration.
(D) immediate transcutaneous pacing.

123. You arrive on scene of a patient who presents in ventricular fibrillation. After immediate defibrillation, no vital signs are obtainable and you note the following rhythm on the monitor:

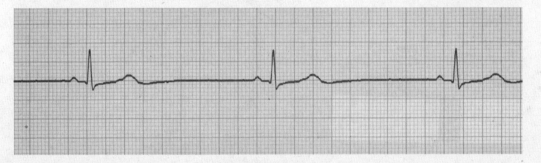

Initial treatment should include
(A) immediate transcutaneous pacing.
(B) atropine 1 mg IVP.
(C) epinephrine 1 mg IVP.
(D) vasopressin 40 units IVP.

124. You have just administered 0.4 mg of sublingual nitroglycerin to a 60-year-old woman with severe chest pain. The patient is receiving high-flow oxygen and has an IV line of normal saline in place. After 5 minutes, the patient states that the pain has not subsided. You should
    (A) repeat the nitroglycerin.
    (B) administer morphine.
    (C) repeat aspirin administration.
    (D) reassess her blood pressure.

125. You are performing CPR on an elderly woman in cardiac arrest. After the patient has been intubated and proper ET tube placement has been confirmed, you should
    (A) perform asynchronous CPR while ventilating the patient at a rate of 8 to 10 breaths/minute.
    (B) pause after 30 compressions so your partner can deliver 2 ventilations.
    (C) administer 2.5 mg of epinephrine via the ET tube and hyperventilate the patient to ensure drug dispersal.
    (D) direct your partner to deliver 1 breath every 3 to 5 seconds.

ANSWERS AND ANSWER EXPLANATIONS

1. **(C)** Arteriosclerosis is a disease of the arterial vessel marked by thickening, hardening, and loss of elasticity in the arterial walls. Atherosclerosis **(A)** is the most common form of arteriosclerosis, usually involving medium-sized and large arteries. Arteriolonecrosis, **(B)** is destruction (necrosis) of the arteriole. Choice **(D)**, angina is chest discomfort associated with a deficiency of oxygen supply to the heart muscle.

2. **(B)** The point of maximal impulse is usually located in the left anterior chest, in the midclavicular line, at the fifth intercostal space. This is an excellent place to auscultate heart sounds and apical pulse.

3. **(B)** Cardiac output is defined as the volume of blood ejected from the left ventricle into the arterial system each minute. Preload **(A)** is defined as the pressure within the ventricles at the end of diastole. Afterload **(C)** is defined as the resistance against which the heart must pump. Stroke volume **(D)** is defined as the amount of blood ejected by the heart in one cardiac contraction.

4. **(D)** Medications with a positive chronotropic effect will increase the heart rate.

5. **(A)** Afterload is defined as the resistance against which the heart must pump. Blood pressure **(B)** is defined as pressure that is exerted on the walls of arteries. Preload **(C)** is defined as the pressure within the ventricles at the end of diastole. Cardiac output **(D)** is defined as the volume of blood ejected from the left ventricle into the arterial system each minute.

6. **(B)** Stroke volume is defined as the amount of blood ejected by the heart in one cardiac contraction. Cardiac output **(A)** is defined as the volume of blood ejected from the left ventricle into the arterial system each minute. Preload **(C)** is defined as the pressure within the ventricles at the end of diastole. Afterload **(D)** is defined as the resistance against which the heart must pump.

7. **(B)** Hypocalcemia results in decreased contractility and increased myocardial irritability. Hypomagnesemia results in increased myocardial irritability.

8. **(D)** The pericardium is the fibroserous sac enclosing the heart that is composed of two layers, the epicardium and the parietal pericardium. The myocardium **(A)** is the middle layer of the walls of the heart. The septum **(B)** is the inner walls of the heart that separate the right and left atria of the heart from the ventricles. The endocardium **(C)** is the innermost layer of the heart.

9. **(C)** Proventil has beta-2-specific properties. This medication can cause cardiac side effects and should be used with caution in patients with heart disease.

10. **(A)** The absence of AMI on the 12-lead doesn't mean that patient isn't having one. It may take hours for changes to appear on the 12-lead. A normal 12-lead ECG should not be used to determine whether a patient should be treated in the field for AMI. You must use clinical judgment to help determine treatment.

11. **(A)** When you are looking for evidence of injury to the heart, you must see it in two or more contiguous leads. For example, lead III is contiguous with leads II and aVF.

12. **(D)** Lead V_6 is contiguous with lead V_5 and lead I. These three leads monitor the lateral wall of the heart and the left ventricle.

13. **(B)** An acute infarction to the inferior wall will present with ST segment elevation in leads II, III, and aVF. **(D)** is incorrect because ST segment depression indicates ischemia and not acute infarction.

14. **(A)** V_3 and V_4 monitor the anterior wall of the myocardium. T-wave inversion indicates ischemia. **(D)** is incorrect because ST segment elevation indicates injury/infarction.

15. **(C)** Infarction often results in the development of a pathological Q wave. A Q wave that is wider than 0.04 second or deeper than one third of the height of the R wave and is present in two or more contiguous leads generally indicates infarction.

16. **(D)** Leads V_1 to V_3 allow you to view the anterior and septal wall of the left ventricle.

17. **(D)** The jugular veins reflect the pressure within systemic circulation. Normally, the jugular veins are not distended in a patient sitting or standing. JVD present at a 45° angle indicates that pressure in the right side of the heart is elevated and indicates right heart compromise. **(B)** is not the best answer because the question does not give you any indication of the patient's respiratory status.

18. **(B)** Fentanyl is quickly becoming the medication of choice for chest pain unrelieved by nitroglycerin because of its rapid onset, relatively short duration, and fewer side effects than morphine.

19. **(D)** In lead II placement, the positive electrode is located on the left leg, the negative electrode on the right shoulder, and the ground on the left shoulder.

20. **(D)** In lead III placement, the positive electrode is located on the left leg, the negative electrode on the left shoulder, and the ground on the right shoulder.

21. **(C)** 0.04 second is measured in each small square on the ECG graph paper. Each large block is 0.20 second.

22. **(D)** Each large block on the ECG graph paper represents 0.20 second. Each small block measures 0.04 second.

23. **(D)** Fundamentals of ECG interpretation tell us that a normal PR interval is 0.12 to 0.20 second.

24. **(D)** Fundamentals of ECG interpretation tell us that the normal duration of a QRS complex is 0.08 to 0.12 second.

25. **(A)** The intrinsic firing rate for a ventricular pacemaker is 20 to 40 beats per minute. The intrinsic firing rate of the SA node (the primary pacemaker of the heart) is 60 to 100 **(C)**. The AV node also has pacemaker ability at a firing rate of 40 to 60 beats per minute **(B)**. There is no normal pacemaker of the heart with a firing rate of 100 to 150 beats per minute.

26. **(D)** The PR interval is the time elapsing between the beginning of the P wave and the beginning of the QRS complex. The normal duration of the PR interval is 0.12 to 0.20 second. The QRS complex **(A)** reflects ventricular depolarization. First-degree heart block **(B)** is an ECG rhythm with a PR interval greater than 0.20 second. The QT interval **(C)** is measured from the beginning of the Q wave to the end of the T wave.

27. **(C)** The return of a cardiac muscle to its resting state is repolarization. Automaticity **(D)** is the ability for certain cardiac cells to initiate impulses spontaneously. Choice **(A)**, synapse, is the junction point of two neurons. Choice **(B)**, depolarization, is the change from the resting potential to a positive charge inside the cardiac cell.

28. **(C)** The normal pacemaker of the heart is the sinoatrial node. The normal firing rate of the SA node is 60–100 beats per minute. The AV node **(A)** is the secondary pacemaker of the heart with a firing rate of 40–60 beats per minute. The third pacemaker of the heart is the Purkinje fibers **(B)** in the ventricles with a firing rate of 20–40 beats per minute. The internodal pathways **(D)** do not have pacemaker capabilities.

29. **(A)** The SA node is located high in the right atrium.

30. **(A)** The Bundle of His does not contain pacemaker capabilities. The normal pacemaker of the heart is the SA node **(C)** with a firing rate of 60–100 beats per minute. The AV node **(D)** is the secondary pacemaker of the heart with a firing rate of 40–60 beats per minute. The third pacemaker of the heart is the Purkinje fibers **(B)** in the ventricles with a firing rate of 20–40 beats per minute.

31. **(B)** The intrinsic firing rate of the AV node is 40–60 beats per minute. The normal pacemaker of the heart is the sinoatrial node with a normal firing rate of 60–100 beats per minute. The third pacemaker of the heart is the Purkinje fibers in the ventricles with a firing rate of 20–40 beats per minute **(A)**. The internodal pathways do not have pacemaker capabilities. **(C)** is incorrect. No normal pacemaker of the heart has a firing rate of 40–80 beats per minute.

32. **(A)** The first component of the ECG is the P wave, which represents depolarization of the atria.

33. **(C)** The QRS complex reflects ventricular depolarization. The Q wave is the first negative deflection after the P wave; the R wave is the first positive deflection after the P wave; and the S wave is the first negative deflection after the R wave. All three waves are not always present.

34. **(D)** The T wave reflects repolarization of the ventricles.

35. **(A)** The PR interval is the time elapsing between the beginning of the P wave and the beginning of the QRS complex **(C)**. The normal duration of the PR interval is 0.12 to 0.20 second. The PR interval represents the time it takes for an electrical impulse to be transmitted from the atria to the ventricles. The T wave **(B)** represents ventricular repolarization. The QRS complex **(C)** reflects ventricular depolarization. The J point **(D)** is found at the junction of the QRS complex and the ST segment.

36. **(C)** The period of the cardiac cycle when stimulation will not produce depolarization is the absolute refractory period. The refractory period **(A)** is a period of time when myocardial cells have not yet completely repolarized and cannot be stimulated again. The relative refractory period **(D)** is a period of time when a significantly strong stimulus may produce depolarization. **(B)** is not a term used in cardiology.

37. **(D)** The period of the cardiac cycle when a significantly strong stimulus may produce depolarization is the relative refractory period. The period of the cardiac cycle when stimulation will not produce depolarization is the absolute refractory period **(C)**. The refractory period **(A)** is a period of time

when myocardial cells have not yet completely repolarized and cannot be stimulated again. (B) is not a term used in cardiology.

38. **(C)** Stimulation of the vagus nerve can occur in many ways. When stimulated, a decrease in heart rate may be observed.

39. **(A)** A rapid heart rate or irregular heartbeat may cause a patient to experience a sensation commonly referred to as palpitations. Another common term to describe this sensation is "fluttering."

40. **(B)** Cardiogenic shock is the most severe form of pump failure that often results in dysrhythmias, hypotension, respiratory failure, and possibly organ failure. The heart rate is initially elevated as the body attempts to compensate for the shock. Hypertension will not be present in cardiogenic shock.

41. **(D)** Left ventricular failure occurs when the heart fails as an effective forward pump, which causes backpressure of blood into pulmonary circulation. When the backpressure becomes high enough, it forces the blood into the capillaries of the alveoli resulting in pulmonary congestion. Adventitious lung sounds such as crackles (rales) are commonly present in left ventricular failure.

42. **(D)** Administration of nitroglycerin gr1/150 sublingual is the only correct choice for this question. Establishing an IV (A) is warranted for a patient complaining of chest pain but the IV should be run at KVO. Administration of Lasix (B) may be appropriate if signs/symptoms of left ventricular failure are present but the dose of 100 mg is excessive. You certainly want to administer oxygen (C) but a high flow rate is recommended to increase oxygen delivery to the myocardium.

43. **(A)** CPAP is the standard of care for respiratory distress secondary to congestive failure and pulmonary edema. (C) is incorrect because these medications should not be administered ahead of oxygen therapy and CPAP. Furosemide and morphine have been moved to the bottom of most CHF protocols or removed entirely.

44. **(B)** Management of cardiogenic shock may include the administration of IV dopamine. Dopamine is a vasopressor that increases cardiac output. You would not want to administer morphine or nitroglycerin (A and C) since they will further lower the blood pressure. An IV at 500 cc/hr (D) is not warranted because administering additional IV fluid to the patient will worsen the condition.

45. **(B)** One bisphasic shock at 120 joules is required upon the diagnosis of ventricular fibrillation. Management of the airway is important, but the airway should be maintained by basic methods until defibrillation is per-

formed. Endotracheal intubation (A) may be attempted after defibrillation. Administration of medications (C and D) is secondary treatment to defibrillation.

46. **(B)** Back and flank pain described as a tearing sensation and a pulsating abdominal mass are classic signs of an abdominal aortic aneurysm. Gentle handling and rapid transport to the hospital are essential once the diagnosis is made. Palpating the mass (A) is contraindicated and may worsen the condition. (C) and (D) are incorrect because there is not enough information given in the scenario to administer any medications.

47. **(D)** Procainamide should be discontinued if the QRS is widened 50% of its original width, the maximum dose is achieved, the arrhythmia is suppressed, or hypotension develops.

48. **(B)** Adenosine is not indicated in the treatment of ventricular fibrillation. It is useful in the treatment of narrow complex tachycardias. Epinephrine, lidocaine, and vasopressin all have indications in the treatment of ventricular fibrillation.

49. **(D)** Paroxysmal supraventricular tachycardia (PSVT) may require synchronized cardioversion, especially if the patient is hemodynamically unstable. Pulseless ventricular tachycardia (A) and ventricular fibrillation (C) require immediate defibrillation, not cardioversion. Synchronized cardioversion is not indicated in pulseless electrical activity, (B).

50. **(B)** ABCs and high-flow oxygen are indicated for this patient and cardioversion needs to be performed because the patient is in ventricular tachycardia *with a pulse*. (A) and (D) are incorrect because this patient should receive cardioversion prior to any administration of medication. (C) is incorrect because Adenocard is not indicated.

51. **(C)** The patient's history should lead you to the conclusion of a vasovagal episode. Having a bowel movement or bearing down to have a bowel movement can stimulate the vagus nerve and slow down the heart rate enough to cause dizziness/syncope. (A), (B), and (D) are incorrect because the scenario did not give you enough information to reach that conclusion.

52. **(C)** Bystander CPR is a courageous effort to save a life and is important in the chain of survival but there are times when bystanders perform CPR inappropriately. As an EMS provider, you must stop bystander CPR and verify a patent airway, the absence of breathing, and pulselessness when you arrive on scene.

53. **(B)** Hyperthermia is not considered a treatable cause of pulseless electrical activity. All of the following are considered treatable causes of PEA: hypov-

olemia, hypoxia, acidosis, hyper/hypokalemia, hypothermia, drug overdose, cardiac tamponade, tension pneumothorax, coronary thrombosis, and pulmonary embolism.

54. **(C)** IV, oxygen, and Adenocard 6 mg rapid IV push are indicated for this patient. Cardioversion **(D)** may be needed if the medication fails to convert the rhythm but is not immediately indicated since the patient lacks serious signs/symptoms of chest pain, dyspnea, or hypotension. Although the items in **(B)** are things you may do for the patient, it is not the best choice. **(A)** is incorrect since you cannot assume this.

55. **(A)** Of the choices listed, nitroglycerin is the best answer since it is indicated for the treatment of chest pain. A fluid bolus **(B)** is not indicated since the patient is not hypotensive and already has evidence of pulmonary congestion (crackles). Atropine **(C)** may be needed if the patient develops unstable signs/symptoms. Transcutaneous pacing **(D)** is not indicated at this point.

56. **(A)** Atropine is indicated for this patient since it appears that he is deteriorating (the BP has dropped and increased pulmonary congestion). At this point, the application of pacing pads to the patient would not be unreasonable in preparation for the possibility of future deterioration of the patient. **(B)** and **(C)** are not indicated for this patient.

57. **(C)** Immediate transcutaneous pacing is required for a hemodynamically unstable (altered LOC, chest pain, dyspnea, hypotension) bradycardic rhythm.

58. **(A)** This rhythm is ventricular fibrillation. Of the choices listed, amiodarone 300 mg is indicated. The dose of lidocaine and procainamide **(B)** and **(C)** are incorrect. Magnesium **(D)** is not indicated.

59. **(A)** If a second dose of amiodarone is needed in the treatment of ventricular fibrillation, the correct dose is 150 mg.

60. **(A)** This is a basic life support question to which you must know the correct answer. If you missed this question, do yourself a favor and review infant, child, and adult CPR prior to taking your certification exam.

61. **(A)** This a basic life support question to which you must know the correct answer. If you missed this question, do yourself a favor and review infant, child, and adult CPR prior to taking your certification test.

62. **(C)** Calcium chloride may be useful in cardiac arrest with known or suspected hyperkalemia. Dialysis patients often suffer from hyperkalemia as a result of their disease process.

63. **(D)** Vasopressin is indicated in ventricular fibrillation at a dose of 40 *units* IV to be administered as a *one-time* dose.

64. **(C)** The maximum amount of procainamide to be administered is 17 mg/kg. The patient's weight is 89.09 kg; 89.09 × 17 equals 1,514 mg maximum dose.

65. **(C)** The initial dose of adenosine is 6 mg. Because the half-life of adenosine is so short, all doses should be administered rapid IV push, immediately followed by a 20 cc bolus of fluid.

66. **(B)** 160–325 mg is the current recommended dose of aspirin for a patient experiencing chest pain/acute coronary syndrome.

67. **(D)** This is a simple math for medication administration question. If you missed this question, a review of math is strongly recommended prior to taking your examination.

68. **(B)** Two grams of lidocaine in 500 cc of solution will provide a mixture of 4 mg/ml. To deliver 2 mg/min using 60 gtt/ml tubing, you need to administer 30 drops per minute.

69. **(D)** The best treatment for a shockable rhythm is defibrillation. If an AED is in the process of delivering a shock, allow it to do so. Removing the AED to apply your own equipment **(C)** will likely cause a delay in this essential treatment.

70. **(A)** The classic description of pain associated with a dissecting aortic aneurysm is a ripping or tearing sensation.

71. **(B)** Vasopressin is indicated only for the management of ventricular fibrillation and pulseless ventricular tachycardia.

72. **(A)** The only correct choice is atropine. Atropine is indicated since the patient presents with chest pain, difficulty breathing, heart rate 42, and BP 76/42. These are considered serious signs and symptoms. A transvenous pacemaker is not utilized in EMS. Having a transcutaneous pacemaker available may be useful if the medication is ineffective, an altered LOC is observed, or the patient deteriorates. **(B)** is incorrect because the patient needs high flow oxygen. **(D)** is incorrect because the dose is wrong.

73. **(C)** Don't overlook the obvious. This question displays the normal values of sinus rhythm.

74. **(D)** This ECG demonstrates a sinus tachycardia.

75. **(C)** This ECG demonstrates atrial fibrillation.

76. **(A)** Treatment for this patient would include oxygen, IV, continued monitoring and observation. Studies have shown that atrial fibrillation can decrease cardiac output as much as 33%. This patient should be transported for evaluation, especially if this rhythm is a new development for the patient. **(B)**, **(C)**, and **(D)** are not indicated in this scenario.

77. **(B)** This ECG demonstrates ventricular tachycardia.

78. **(A)** Treatment of this unstable patient is synchronous cardioversion. Defibrillation **(B)** is not indicated since the patient has a pulse. If this patient were pulseless, the treatment would include defibrillation. **(C)** and **(D)** are not indicated for this patient.

79. **(A)** This ECG demonstrates a sinus rhythm with PACs.

80. **(A)** Treatment for this patient includes Adenocard 6 mg IVP since chest pain is present. This scenario does not present an unstable patient and therefore cardioversion **(B)** is not indicated. Although you will continue to assess and monitor this patient, **(C)** is not the best choice since chest pain is present and Adenocard is indicated. **(D)** is not indicated.

81. **(A)** 17 mcg/kg is incorrect because procainamide is delivered in mg/kg.

82. **(D)** Of the choices listed, oxygen is the only appropriate treatment. Nitroglycerin and aspirin **(A)** and **(C)** are not indicated since the scenario does not include a complaint of chest pain. Procardia **(B)** is contraindicated.

83. **(A)** Adenocard is indicated for the treatment of a narrow complex tachycardia.

84. **(A)** The first medication to be delivered after defibrillating pulseless ventricular tachycardia is epinephrine or vasopressin.

85. **(C)** Vasopressin is indicated in the management of ventricular fibrillation and pulseless ventricular tachycardia.

86. **(D)** A single dose of 40 units IV is the recommended dose of vasopressin.

87. **(B)** Amiodarone has not been approved to be administered via the endotracheal route.

88. **(B)** The correct second dose of Amiodarone for a patient in v fib is 150 mg IVP.

89. **(C)** This is a basic life support question. If you missed this question, do yourself a favor and review infant, child, and adult CPR prior to taking your certification test.

90. **(A)** Acute coronary syndrome is defined as a sudden ischemic disorder of the heart. If you are not familiar with this terminology, it is strongly recommended that you review Section Four of the American Heart Association ACLS Providers Manual.

91. **(C)** Hypoglycemia is not considered an anginal equivalent.

92. **(D)** All of the signs and symptoms are considered atypical presentation of myocardial ischemia.

93. **(C)** Nitroglycerin is a vasodilator, works against vasospasm, and decreases preload. It does not have an effect on afterload.

94. **(C)** The classic signs/symptoms in this scenario that should lead you to suspect congestive heart failure in this patient are "He was awakened from his sleep with shortness of breath," and he has signs of pulmonary congestion (crackles) present.

95. **(A)** Of the choices listed, preparation for intubation is the only correct answer. **(C)** is incorrect because CPAP should not be used in a lethargic patient.

96. **(C)** Treatment for this unstable patient is synchronous cardioversion since the patient has a pulse. If this patient was pulseless, the treatment would include defibrillation **(B)**. Lidocaine **(A)** is not *initial* treatment but may be given secondary to cardioversion. **(D)** is not indicated.

97. **(D)** Observation is the only correct choice. **(A)** is incorrect because the patient is not hemodynamically unstable. **(C)** is incorrect because the dose listed is incorrect.

98. **(D)** Immediate defibrillation is indicated for the treatment of ventricular fibrillation.

99. **(A)** Atropine is the correct choice. **(B)** is incorrect because the dose for vasopressin is incorrect.

100. **(C)** Since the patient's presentation is considered stable, a vagal maneuver is indicated.

101. **(D)** Immediate transcutaneous pacing is indicated for type two second-degree AV block and third-degree AV block when accompanied with symptoms.

102. **(B)** Milliamps should be increased until mechanical capture is obtained.

103. **(A)** This rhythm indicates a paced rhythm with 1:1 capture. The patient should receive oxygen, IV, monitor, and continued observation. Neither lidocaine nor cardioversion **(B)** and **(D)** are indicated for this rhythm and nitroglycerin and ASA **(C)** are not indicated for the present complaints.

104. **(B)** Four hours of chest pain with no relief after 12 nitroglycerin is best classified as unstable angina. Stable angina **(A)** is somewhat predictable in onset, severity, character, and response to therapy. Prinzmetal's (AKA vasospastic angina) **(C)** and **(D)** is angina caused by decreased blood flow due to spasm of a vessel.

105. **(C)** A severe "tearing sensation" epigastric pain that radiates into the back and shoulders is the classic description of pain often associated with an aortic aneurysm.

106. **(C)** Dopamine at 1–2 mcg/kg/min administration causes renal artery dilation to occur. At 2–10 mcg/kg/min, it primarily affects beta receptors. At 10–15 mcg/kg/min, it primarily affects both alpha and beta receptors. At 15–20 mcg/kg/min it primarily affects alpha receptors.

107. **(B)** Vasopressin is indicated in ventricular fibrillation at a dose of 40 *units* IV to be administered as a *one-time* dose.

108. **(B)** Sodium bicarbonate has been in use for a long time. Current dosing instructions include 1 mEq/kg.

109. **(A)** Dopamine is a vasopressor primarily used by EMS to improve cardiac output in cardiogenic shock. A side effect of dopamine administration is an increased oxygen demand and workload on the heart. Therefore, dopamine must be used with caution when cardiac ischemia is suspected.

110. **(B)** The second dose of amiodarone for the treatment of ventricular fibrillation is 150 mg.

111. **(B)** A side effect of amiodarone administration is vasodilation and hypotension. This is mainly the reason amiodarone is to be administered slow IV. Rapid IV administration of amiodarone may produce profound hypotension.

112. **(D)** Lidocaine is contraindicated in severe degrees of SA, AV, or intraventricular blocks because it may produce serious ventricular dysrhythmias or develop into complete heart block.

113. **(B)** Nitroglycerin is not indicated for this patient because of the presence of hypotension.

114. **(C)** Prehospital indications for the administration of sodium bicarbonate include tricyclic antidepressant overdose, hyperkalemia, and preexisting or suspected acidosis.

Questions 115 to 119 are basic life support questions. If you miss any of these questions, it is essential to review basic CPR prior to taking your exam.

115. **(C)** Looking, listening, and feeling the airflow through the victim's nose or mouth.

116. **(D)** Full chest recoil between compressions.

117. **(C)** 30 compressions to 2 ventilations.

118. **(C)** 30 compressions to 2 ventilations.

119. **(C)** 100 times per minute.

120. **(C)** Transport for evaluation must be considered for this patient. A bradycardic rate of 48 while mowing the lawn on a hot August day should be a concern. With the presence of chest pain, you should suspect an underlying cardiac origin and transport.

121. **(D)** If a reversible cause of asystole is not rapidly identified and the patient fails to respond to treatment, termination of resuscitation efforts may be considered.

122. **(D)** This rhythm is complete heart block. With the presence of serious signs/symptoms, immediate transcutaneous pacing is indicated.

123. **(C)** Epinephrine is the first medication to be administered in the pulseless electrical activity algorithm.

124. **(D)** As simple as it sounds, reassessment of the blood pressure in between doses of nitroglycerin is the correct choice.

125. **(A)** After an advanced airway is placed, "cycles" of CPR are no longer delivered. Give continuous chest compressions without pauses for breaths. Give 8 to 10 breaths per minute.

Notes

Notes

Medical Emergencies

 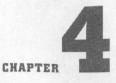

Medical emergencies is a generic title for literally thousands of conditions. This chapter is focused on assessment, recognitions, and treatment of the more common medical emergencies encountered by EMS providers. Topics include

- Respiratory
- Neurology
- Endocrinology
- Allergies/Anaphylaxis
- Gastroenterology
- Urology
- Environmental
- Behavioral
- Toxicology

All ECG rhythm strips used in this chapter are six-second strips.

Answer Sheet

CHAPTER 4—MEDICAL EMERGENCIES

1 Ⓐ Ⓑ Ⓒ Ⓓ	39 Ⓐ Ⓑ Ⓒ Ⓓ	77 Ⓐ Ⓑ Ⓒ Ⓓ	115 Ⓐ Ⓑ Ⓒ Ⓓ
2 Ⓐ Ⓑ Ⓒ Ⓓ	40 Ⓐ Ⓑ Ⓒ Ⓓ	78 Ⓐ Ⓑ Ⓒ Ⓓ	116 Ⓐ Ⓑ Ⓒ Ⓓ
3 Ⓐ Ⓑ Ⓒ Ⓓ	41 Ⓐ Ⓑ Ⓒ Ⓓ	79 Ⓐ Ⓑ Ⓒ Ⓓ	117 Ⓐ Ⓑ Ⓒ Ⓓ
4 Ⓐ Ⓑ Ⓒ Ⓓ	42 Ⓐ Ⓑ Ⓒ Ⓓ	80 Ⓐ Ⓑ Ⓒ Ⓓ	118 Ⓐ Ⓑ Ⓒ Ⓓ
5 Ⓐ Ⓑ Ⓒ Ⓓ	43 Ⓐ Ⓑ Ⓒ Ⓓ	81 Ⓐ Ⓑ Ⓒ Ⓓ	119 Ⓐ Ⓑ Ⓒ Ⓓ
6 Ⓐ Ⓑ Ⓒ Ⓓ	44 Ⓐ Ⓑ Ⓒ Ⓓ	82 Ⓐ Ⓑ Ⓒ Ⓓ	120 Ⓐ Ⓑ Ⓒ Ⓓ
7 Ⓐ Ⓑ Ⓒ Ⓓ	45 Ⓐ Ⓑ Ⓒ Ⓓ	83 Ⓐ Ⓑ Ⓒ Ⓓ	121 Ⓐ Ⓑ Ⓒ Ⓓ
8 Ⓐ Ⓑ Ⓒ Ⓓ	46 Ⓐ Ⓑ Ⓒ Ⓓ	84 Ⓐ Ⓑ Ⓒ Ⓓ	122 Ⓐ Ⓑ Ⓒ Ⓓ
9 Ⓐ Ⓑ Ⓒ Ⓓ	47 Ⓐ Ⓑ Ⓒ Ⓓ	85 Ⓐ Ⓑ Ⓒ Ⓓ	123 Ⓐ Ⓑ Ⓒ Ⓓ
10 Ⓐ Ⓑ Ⓒ Ⓓ	48 Ⓐ Ⓑ Ⓒ Ⓓ	86 Ⓐ Ⓑ Ⓒ Ⓓ	124 Ⓐ Ⓑ Ⓒ Ⓓ
11 Ⓐ Ⓑ Ⓒ Ⓓ	49 Ⓐ Ⓑ Ⓒ Ⓓ	87 Ⓐ Ⓑ Ⓒ Ⓓ	125 Ⓐ Ⓑ Ⓒ Ⓓ
12 Ⓐ Ⓑ Ⓒ Ⓓ	50 Ⓐ Ⓑ Ⓒ Ⓓ	88 Ⓐ Ⓑ Ⓒ Ⓓ	126 Ⓐ Ⓑ Ⓒ Ⓓ
13 Ⓐ Ⓑ Ⓒ Ⓓ	51 Ⓐ Ⓑ Ⓒ Ⓓ	89 Ⓐ Ⓑ Ⓒ Ⓓ	127 Ⓐ Ⓑ Ⓒ Ⓓ
14 Ⓐ Ⓑ Ⓒ Ⓓ	52 Ⓐ Ⓑ Ⓒ Ⓓ	90 Ⓐ Ⓑ Ⓒ Ⓓ	128 Ⓐ Ⓑ Ⓒ Ⓓ
15 Ⓐ Ⓑ Ⓒ Ⓓ	53 Ⓐ Ⓑ Ⓒ Ⓓ	91 Ⓐ Ⓑ Ⓒ Ⓓ	129 Ⓐ Ⓑ Ⓒ Ⓓ
16 Ⓐ Ⓑ Ⓒ Ⓓ	54 Ⓐ Ⓑ Ⓒ Ⓓ	92 Ⓐ Ⓑ Ⓒ Ⓓ	130 Ⓐ Ⓑ Ⓒ Ⓓ
17 Ⓐ Ⓑ Ⓒ Ⓓ	55 Ⓐ Ⓑ Ⓒ Ⓓ	93 Ⓐ Ⓑ Ⓒ Ⓓ	131 Ⓐ Ⓑ Ⓒ Ⓓ
18 Ⓐ Ⓑ Ⓒ Ⓓ	56 Ⓐ Ⓑ Ⓒ Ⓓ	94 Ⓐ Ⓑ Ⓒ Ⓓ	132 Ⓐ Ⓑ Ⓒ Ⓓ
19 Ⓐ Ⓑ Ⓒ Ⓓ	57 Ⓐ Ⓑ Ⓒ Ⓓ	95 Ⓐ Ⓑ Ⓒ Ⓓ	133 Ⓐ Ⓑ Ⓒ Ⓓ
20 Ⓐ Ⓑ Ⓒ Ⓓ	58 Ⓐ Ⓑ Ⓒ Ⓓ	96 Ⓐ Ⓑ Ⓒ Ⓓ	134 Ⓐ Ⓑ Ⓒ Ⓓ
21 Ⓐ Ⓑ Ⓒ Ⓓ	59 Ⓐ Ⓑ Ⓒ Ⓓ	97 Ⓐ Ⓑ Ⓒ Ⓓ	135 Ⓐ Ⓑ Ⓒ Ⓓ
22 Ⓐ Ⓑ Ⓒ Ⓓ	60 Ⓐ Ⓑ Ⓒ Ⓓ	98 Ⓐ Ⓑ Ⓒ Ⓓ	136 Ⓐ Ⓑ Ⓒ Ⓓ
23 Ⓐ Ⓑ Ⓒ Ⓓ	61 Ⓐ Ⓑ Ⓒ Ⓓ	99 Ⓐ Ⓑ Ⓒ Ⓓ	137 Ⓐ Ⓑ Ⓒ Ⓓ
24 Ⓐ Ⓑ Ⓒ Ⓓ	62 Ⓐ Ⓑ Ⓒ Ⓓ	100 Ⓐ Ⓑ Ⓒ Ⓓ	138 Ⓐ Ⓑ Ⓒ Ⓓ
25 Ⓐ Ⓑ Ⓒ Ⓓ	63 Ⓐ Ⓑ Ⓒ Ⓓ	101 Ⓐ Ⓑ Ⓒ Ⓓ	139 Ⓐ Ⓑ Ⓒ Ⓓ
26 Ⓐ Ⓑ Ⓒ Ⓓ	64 Ⓐ Ⓑ Ⓒ Ⓓ	102 Ⓐ Ⓑ Ⓒ Ⓓ	140 Ⓐ Ⓑ Ⓒ Ⓓ
27 Ⓐ Ⓑ Ⓒ Ⓓ	65 Ⓐ Ⓑ Ⓒ Ⓓ	103 Ⓐ Ⓑ Ⓒ Ⓓ	141 Ⓐ Ⓑ Ⓒ Ⓓ
28 Ⓐ Ⓑ Ⓒ Ⓓ	66 Ⓐ Ⓑ Ⓒ Ⓓ	104 Ⓐ Ⓑ Ⓒ Ⓓ	142 Ⓐ Ⓑ Ⓒ Ⓓ
29 Ⓐ Ⓑ Ⓒ Ⓓ	67 Ⓐ Ⓑ Ⓒ Ⓓ	105 Ⓐ Ⓑ Ⓒ Ⓓ	143 Ⓐ Ⓑ Ⓒ Ⓓ
30 Ⓐ Ⓑ Ⓒ Ⓓ	68 Ⓐ Ⓑ Ⓒ Ⓓ	106 Ⓐ Ⓑ Ⓒ Ⓓ	144 Ⓐ Ⓑ Ⓒ Ⓓ
31 Ⓐ Ⓑ Ⓒ Ⓓ	69 Ⓐ Ⓑ Ⓒ Ⓓ	107 Ⓐ Ⓑ Ⓒ Ⓓ	145 Ⓐ Ⓑ Ⓒ Ⓓ
32 Ⓐ Ⓑ Ⓒ Ⓓ	70 Ⓐ Ⓑ Ⓒ Ⓓ	108 Ⓐ Ⓑ Ⓒ Ⓓ	146 Ⓐ Ⓑ Ⓒ Ⓓ
33 Ⓐ Ⓑ Ⓒ Ⓓ	71 Ⓐ Ⓑ Ⓒ Ⓓ	109 Ⓐ Ⓑ Ⓒ Ⓓ	147 Ⓐ Ⓑ Ⓒ Ⓓ
34 Ⓐ Ⓑ Ⓒ Ⓓ	72 Ⓐ Ⓑ Ⓒ Ⓓ	110 Ⓐ Ⓑ Ⓒ Ⓓ	148 Ⓐ Ⓑ Ⓒ Ⓓ
35 Ⓐ Ⓑ Ⓒ Ⓓ	73 Ⓐ Ⓑ Ⓒ Ⓓ	111 Ⓐ Ⓑ Ⓒ Ⓓ	149 Ⓐ Ⓑ Ⓒ Ⓓ
36 Ⓐ Ⓑ Ⓒ Ⓓ	74 Ⓐ Ⓑ Ⓒ Ⓓ	112 Ⓐ Ⓑ Ⓒ Ⓓ	150 Ⓐ Ⓑ Ⓒ Ⓓ
37 Ⓐ Ⓑ Ⓒ Ⓓ	75 Ⓐ Ⓑ Ⓒ Ⓓ	113 Ⓐ Ⓑ Ⓒ Ⓓ	
38 Ⓐ Ⓑ Ⓒ Ⓓ	76 Ⓐ Ⓑ Ⓒ Ⓓ	114 Ⓐ Ⓑ Ⓒ Ⓓ	

1. You receive a call to the home of a 66-year-old male with a complaint of weakness. The patient is cooperative but continues to ask you the same questions over and over again. You are concerned because he has developed increased confusion over the past five minutes and is now diaphoretic. Your next action is to
   (A) further assess for facial droop, drooling, and motor weakness.
   (B) further assess to determine if a head injury has occurred.
   (C) establish an IV and obtain a blood sample for a blood glucose test.
   (D) administer nitroglycerin and baby ASA for atypical presentation of myocardial infarction.

2. You find a morbidly obese 42-year-old patient lying supine in his bed. He is in marked respiratory distress and is able to speak only in two-word sentences. What should you do FIRST?
   (A) Begin assisting his ventilations.
   (B) Assess his oxygen saturation level.
   (C) Administer a beta-2 agonist drug.
   (D) Sit him up or place him on his side.

3. The pathophysiology of Type II diabetes mellitus includes, polydipsia, polyuria, and _____ .
   (A) polyphagia
   (B) polycythemia
   (C) alkalosis
   (D) glycosuria

4. When the body is not able to use glucose as a primary source of energy
   (A) adipose cells begin breaking down resulting in hyperglycemia.
   (B) adipose cells begin breaking down resulting in hypoglycemia.
   (C) adipose cells begin breaking down resulting in hyperinsulinism.
   (D) adipose cells begin breaking down resulting in ketoacidosis.

5. Signs and symptoms of _____ include agitation, emotional changes, insomnia, heat intolerance, weight loss, and exophthalmos.
   (A) myxedema
   (B) malaise
   (C) Graves' disease
   (D) hypothyroidism

6. A male patient has ingested 30 levothyroxine that belonged to his mother. You recognize this medication as a thyroid replacement hormone. You attach the ECG monitor and observe a sinus tachycardia of 140 with a corresponding pulse rate. Treatment would include
   (A) expedited transport for definitive care.
   (B) Adenocard 6 mg rapid IVP.
   (C) Adenocard 12 mg rapid IVP.
   (D) verapamil 2.5 mg slow IVP.

7. A patient with Cushing's syndrome would MOST likely present with
   (A) ketoacidosis.
   (B) hypoglycemia.
   (C) decreased urination.
   (D) acute hyperactivity.

8. You are caring for a 78-year-old female patient who has a long history of hyperadrenalism (Cushing's syndrome). She is complaining of left side weakness. You are assigned to establish an IV line and obtain a blood sample for blood glucose testing. You should
   (A) take great care with venipuncture in this patient because hyperadrenalism leads to easy bruising and a delay in healing.
   (B) refuse to establish intravenous access because the veins are fragile and the skin is paper thin.
   (C) not bother checking a blood glucose level because Cushing's syndrome is always associated with hyperglycemia.
   (D) None of the above are correct.

9. Hyperadrenalism is
   (A) associated with a high incident of atherosclerosis including hypertension and stroke.
   (B) associated with low metabolism rate and poor organ function.
   (C) associated with thyrotoxicosis.
   (D) associated with an increased insulin production.

10. A patient experiencing Addisonian crisis may display which of the following signs/symptoms?
    (A) Increased appetite, hypoglycemia, hyperthermia
    (B) Extreme hypertension, elevated temperature, vomiting
    (C) Cardiovascular collapse, hypotension, hypoglycemia
    (D) Coma secondary to hypothyroidism

11. You have a patient who presents with a whole body rash. There is no complaint of shortness of breath. Which of the following history findings lead you to conclude that the rash is the result of a delayed hypersensitivity reaction?
    (A) History of eating shellfish 30 minutes ago
    (B) History of taking a new medication for the past seven days
    (C) History of insect sting last summer
    (D) History of chlamydia

Questions 12 and 13 are based on the following scenario:
You are called to an elementary school. On arrival, you are directed to a teacher. The class is holding a birthday party for Austin, who turned 10 today. Austin's mom baked brownies for the party that contained nuts.

12. The teacher is allergic to nuts. She ate the brownies five minutes ago. She complains of tightness in her chest that is making it difficult to breathe. She is not able to talk in full sentences. Given this information, you suspect the patient is experiencing
    (A) a simple allergic reaction.
    (B) a severe allergic reaction.
    (C) sensitization.
    (D) delayed hypersensitivity.

13. Her respiratory distress is becoming worse. Her blood pressure is 74/48, pulse 140, respirations 40. You decide to administer epinephrine. The correct dose and route are
    (A) 0.01–0.03 mg of 1:1,000 solution SQ.
    (B) 0.3–0.5 cc of 1:10,000 solution IV.
    (C) 3–5 ml of 1:10,000 solution IV.
    (D) 0.1–0.3 mg of 1:1,000 solution SQ.

---

14. Online medical control orders you to administer 100 mg of diphenhydramine (Benadryl) IV to a patient with a severe allergic reaction. You would
    (A) administer it slowly since hypotension and sedation may result.
    (B) administer it rapidly to prevent vomiting and headache.
    (C) ask medical control to repeat the dosage because you question 100 mg as being excessive.
    (D) administer it slowly to prevent burning at the injection site.

15. Maroon or tarry-colored stool indicates:
    (A) peritonitis.
    (B) bowel obstruction.
    (C) the presence of partially digested blood.
    (D) a normal finding in alcoholism.

Questions 16–18 are based on the following scenario:
You arrive on scene of a 30-year-old male lying on the ground. According to a bystander, the patient was on top of a ladder changing a light bulb. After he stuck his hand in the light fixture, he was attacked by yellow jackets that had a nest in the fixture. The patient then jumped from the top of the ladder to escape the bees. You estimate his fall to the ground to be 8 feet. He has numerous yellow jacket stings on his left arm and neck.

16. The patient is unconscious and unresponsive. As you assess his airway and breathing, you observe a respiratory rate of 8 per minute with deep gasping respirations, accessory muscle use, and obvious inspiratory stridor with each breath. Management of this patient's airway would include
    (A) c-spine immobilization, oral pharyngeal airway insertion, and high-flow oxygen by nonrebreather mask.
    (B) beginning bag-valve mask ventilations with supplemental oxygen.
    (C) c-spine immobilization, assist ventilations, immediate endotracheal intubation.
    (D) bag-valve mask ventilation with high-flow oxygen at a rate of 24 per minute.

17. Assessment of the chest reveals no obvious trauma. You note equal but distant lung sounds with wheezing on auscultation. You suspect the respiratory distress to be from
    (A) tension pneumothorax.
    (B) hemothorax.
    (C) bronchial constriction secondary to anaphylactic reaction.
    (D) early pneumothorax.

18. You are unable to obtain IV access. Treatment for this patient would include
    (A) immediate chest decompression.
    (B) epinephrine 1:1,000 solution 3–5 ml SQ.
    (C) lidocaine 1 mg/kg IVP.
    (D) epinephrine 1:1,000 solution 0.3–0.5 mg SQ.

---

19. Urticaria is defined as
    (A) nausea, vomiting, and diarrhea associated with allergic reactions.
    (B) raised areas or wheals on the skin due to histamine release.
    (C) release of mast cells that cause bronchial constriction.
    (D) edema of the head, neck, and face associated with severe allergic reaction.

20. You need to administer epinephrine to a 26-year-old male who is short of breath after receiving radiologic contrast material. The subcutaneous dose is
    (A) 0.1–0.3 mg 1:1,000 solution.
    (B) 0.1–0.3 mg 1:10,000 solution.
    (C) 0.5–1.0 mg 1:1,000 solution.
    (D) 0.3–0.5 mg 1:1,000 solution.

21. A sharp type of pain that travels along a definitive neural route is termed
    (A) peritonitis.
    (B) somatic pain.
    (C) referred pain.
    (D) visceral pain.

22. Dull, poorly localized pain that originates in the walls of the hollow organs is termed
    (A) peritonitis.
    (B) somatic pain.
    (C) referred pain.
    (D) visceral pain.

23. Pain that originates in a region other than where it is felt is known as
    (A) peritonitis.
    (B) somatic pain.
    (C) referred pain.
    (D) visceral pain.

24. In a patient with abdominal pain, assessment of the abdomen should be performed in the following order:
    (A) Auscultate, palpate, inspect, percuss
    (B) Inspect, percuss, palpate, auscultate
    (C) Inspect, auscultate, palpate, percuss
    (D) Inspect, auscultate, percuss, palpate

Questions 25 and 26 are based on the following scenario:
You are called for a 62-year-old male with a complaint of severe abdominal pain. He is lying as still as possible in his bed.

25. Upon inspection of the abdomen, you find ecchymosis in the periumbilical area. This is known as
    (A) Cullen's sign.
    (B) Grey-Turner sign.
    (C) peritonitis.
    (D) Mallory-Weiss sign.

26. This assessment finding may indicate
    (A) ascites.
    (B) intraabdominal hemorrhage.
    (C) dissecting aortic aneurysm.
    (D) acute appendicitis.

---

27. You respond to a 21-year-old male with a complaint of vomiting after he drank an excessive amount of alcohol. He is alert, oriented, and experiencing excessive dry heaves at this time. You note the presence of specks of blood on the toilet. He has no history of GI problems and takes no medications. You suspect the bleeding is
    (A) caused by acute gastritis.
    (B) the result of a Mallory-Weiss tear.
    (C) caused by acute peptic ulcer disease.
    (D) caused by acute duodenitis.

28. A patient with severe vomiting presents with the scleras of his eyes dramatically blood red. This is most likely the result of
    (A) hyphema.
    (B) subconjunctival hemorrhage.
    (C) conjunctivitis.
    (D) blunt trauma.

29. You are ordered by medical control to administer Phenergan (promethazine) to a severely nauseated patient. The proper dose range and route should be
    (A) 12.5 to 25 mg IV or deep IM.
    (B) 12.5 to 25 mg SQ, IV or deep IM.
    (C) 25 to 50 mg IV or deep IM.
    (D) 25 mg IV only; IM injection of this medication is not recommended.

30. Ecchymosis in the flank area associated with intraabdominal hemorrhage is known as
    (A) peritonitis.
    (B) Cullen's sign.
    (C) Mallory-Weiss sign.
    (D) Grey-Turner's sign.

Questions 31–34 are based on the following scenario:
You are called to the residence of a 58-year-old male. He is vomiting over the side of the front porch when you arrive. This patient has a history of alcoholism and liver cirrhosis.

31. The patient is conscious but slow to respond and appears highly intoxicated. He asks for your help and falls to the floor. His appearance is pale and diaphoretic with a blood pressure of 90/64, pulse 144, respirations of 36. You note that the porch is covered in coffee-ground emesis. This patient is most likely suffering from
    (A) Mallory-Weiss tear.
    (B) ruptured esophageal varices.
    (C) acute portal hypertension.
    (D) acute abdominal aortic aneurysm rupture.

32. His appearance and vital signs indicate
    (A) acute withdrawal from alcohol.
    (B) shock.
    (C) acute alcohol intoxication.
    (D) alcohol psychosis.

33. Treatment for this patient should include
    (A) close monitoring of airway patency to prevent aspiration, administration of Phenergan to control emesis.
    (B) close monitoring of airway patency, administration of supplemental oxygen, establishing intravenous access, and treatment for shock.
    (C) administering supplemental oxygen, administration of Phenergan to control emesis, and treatment for shock.
    (D) monitoring airway, administering oxygen 3 to 6 liters nasal cannula, transport for alcohol detoxification.

34. During transport to the hospital, your patient has several additional episodes of vomiting. It starts as coffee-ground emesis that quickly changes to bright red blood. He is less responsive with intermediate periods of syncope. Blood pressure is 82/64, pulse 148, respirations 40. You know that
    (A) his change in mental status is secondary to the effects of the alcohol.
    (B) his vital signs and change in mental status indicate decompensated shock.
    (C) his condition is serious and rapid transport is necessary.
    (D) Both B and C are correct.

35. You respond to a local physician's office. You are instructed to assist the physician in performing rapid sequence intubation. You should administer _____ of succinylcholine.
    (A) 0.5–1.0 mg/kg
    (B) 1.5–2.0 mg/kg
    (C) 25 mg
    (D) 100 mg

36. If Succinylcholine is supplied 20 mg/ml, how much medication would you administer to a 186 pound patient?
    (A) 25 mg
    (B) 100 mg
    (C) 125 mg
    (D) 250 mg

37. _____ is an idiopathic inflammatory bowel disorder associated with the small intestine.
    (A) Inguinal hernia
    (B) Crohn's disease
    (C) Diverticulitis
    (D) Ulcerative colitis

38. Small outpouchings of mucosal and submucosal tissue that push through the outermost layer of the intestine is known as
    (A) Crohn's disease.
    (B) inguinal hernia.
    (C) ulcerative colitis.
    (D) diverticulitis.

Questions 39 and 40 are based on the following scenario:

You are assessing a patient with acute right lower quadrant pain. You suspect acute appendicitis.

39. A common site of pain from appendicitis located one to two inches above the anterior iliac crest in a direct line with the umbilicus is known as
    (A) the volvulus point.
    (B) McBurney's point.
    (C) Murphy's sign.
    (D) Grey-Turner's sign.

40. The presence of rebound tenderness in this patient represents
    (A) peritoneal irritation.
    (B) guarding.
    (C) rupture.
    (D) strangulation.

Questions 41–44 are based on the following scenario:
Your patient states that he has experienced right upper quadrant pain and right shoulder pain for the last seven days.

41. The patient is pale, diaphoretic, and in obvious discomfort. He has a bounding pulse rate of 132. He states that this episode of pain began after eating fried onion rings with hot mustard sauce. You suspect his elevated heart rate is caused by
    (A) acute peritonitis.
    (B) stress response to the body and sympathetic nervous system activation.
    (C) an allergic reaction to the mustard.
    (D) acute pancreatitis.

42. You notice that he has pain with palpation under the right costal margin. This is known as
    (A) McBurney's point.
    (B) Murphy's sign.
    (C) Grey-Turner's sign.
    (D) Cullen's sign.

43. With the information gathered, you suspect
    (A) pancreatitis.
    (B) appendicitis.
    (C) cholecystitis.
    (D) diverticulitis.

44. The patient's BP is 188/102, pulse 136, respirations 26. He complains of increased right upper quadrant pain and nausea. Pain medication is indicated. The correct choice of medication for this patient is
    (A) morphine 2–10 mg IV titrated for pain relief.
    (B) Demerol 25–50 mg IV titrated for pain relief.
    (C) fentanyl 25–50 mg IV one time only.
    (D) Nubain 25 mg IV with additional 12.5 mg if needed.

Questions 45 and 46 are based on the following scenario:

A 39-year-old male patient is lying on a couch, covered with several blankets. He has a garbage can next to him that has a small amount of vomitus in it. He has a past medical history of alcoholism.

45. The patient complains of severe epigastric pain that radiates into his back and shoulders. His abdomen is softly distended and he will not allow you to palpate it due to the pain. He states that he took his temperature 30 minutes ago and it was 104.2°F. BP is 86/42, pulse 138, respirations 20. You suspect the patient is suffering from
    (A) peritonitis.
    (B) pancreatitis.
    (C) cholecystitis.
    (D) diverticulitis.

46. You suspect his vital signs are a result of
    (A) hypovolemia from excessive vomiting.
    (B) normal response to infection and hyperpyrexia.
    (C) septic shock from the disease process.
    (D) Both A and C are correct.

---

47. You arrive on scene of a 54-year-old old female patient who is unable to urinate. She states that she had outpatient surgery in which she received anesthesia. She presents in severe discomfort and has a firmly distended bladder that is noticeable on inspection of the abdomen. This patient's situation is

    (A) a true medical emergency.
    (B) does not require ambulance transportation to the hospital.
    (C) requires the administration of Demerol for pain management.
    (D) Both A and C are correct.

Questions 48 and 49 are based on the following scenario:

You respond to the local college campus soccer field for a 20-year-old female patient with a complaint of severe muscle cramps. The temperature is 88°F with high humidity. The patient had just finished a strenuous workout when the cramps began. Her skin is hot to touch and she is sweating profusely.

48. You suspect this patient is suffering
    (A) heatstroke.
    (B) heat exhaustion.
    (C) heat cramps.
    (D) exercise-induced fatigue.

49. Treatment should include
    (A) oral hydration if the patient is able to take fluids.
    (B) two large-bore IVs of normal saline wide open.
    (C) initiating rapid active cooling.
    (D) Both A and C are correct.

Questions 50–53 are based on the following scenario:

Your ambulance is assigned to stand by at a building fire. The outside temperature is 103°F and the firefighters are wearing full protective clothing. Approximately 30 minutes into the incident, a firefighter has collapsed and you are assigned to care for him.

50. The patient is a 36-year-old male in good physical condition. He appears anxious and complains of nausea and a headache. He is sweating profusely with cool clammy skin. BP is 116/48, radial pulse is 150 and weak, respirations are 36 and shallow, temperature is 101.2°F. This patient's signs/symptoms indicate
    (A) heatstroke.
    (B) heat exhaustion.
    (C) heat stress.
    (D) heat fatigue.

51. Treatment for this patient should include all of the following except
    (A) removing clothing.
    (B) establishing IV of normal saline.
    (C) placing in air conditioning.
    (D) administering salt tablets.

52. The patient is now apprehensive. Reassessment reveals a BP of 78/30, pulse 154, respirations 36 and shallow. You are unable to take another temperature because he is not cooperating. His skin is extremely hot to touch and he has stopped sweating. Online medical control has requested that you start rapid active cooling. This can be achieved by
    (A) covering the patient in a sheet that has been soaked in tepid water.
    (B) placing several ice packs under the arms, in the groin, and on the head.
    (C) cold water immersion.
    (D) covering the patient in a sheet that has been soaked in ice water.

53. Which statement is false regarding overcooling of a heatstroke patient?
    (A) It may cause a reflex hypothermia.
    (B) Shivering may result which can lead to a rise in core temperature.
    (C) Body temperature must be lowered immediately with heatstroke and over-cooling is not a concern.
    (D) 102°F should be used as a target temperature to prevent overcooling.

54. Hypothermia is the result of
    (A) an increase in heat loss.
    (B) a decrease in heat production.
    (C) vasodilatation.
    (D) Both A and B are correct.

Questions 55–58 are based on the following scenario:

You are called by the local police department to help search for an elderly man with Alzheimer's disease who wandered away from his home. It is 11:30 P.M. and he has been missing for three hours. It is 38°F outside with a light drizzle. The man is wearing pajamas and slippers.

55. At 4:30 A.M. the patient is located lying behind a pile of wood, five blocks from his home. He is unconscious, unresponsive, apneic, and pulseless. His skin is cold to the touch and his muscles are rigid. His core body temperature is 89.6°F (32°C). Initial treatment should include
    (A) CPR.
    (B) establishing intravenous access with warm normal saline.
    (C) starting passive rewarming.
    (D) placing in a Trendelenburg position.

56. You attach the ECG monitor and observe the following rhythm.

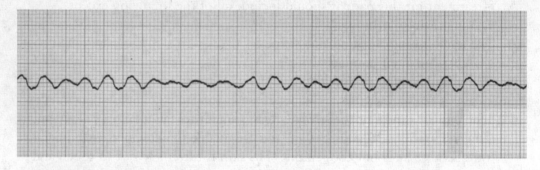

    Treatment should include
    (A) none until the core temperature is 90°F.
    (B) immediate defibrillation.
    (C) avoiding rough movement and excessive activity.
    (D) Both A and C are correct.

57. You are considering the administration of cardiac medication to this patient. Which statement is true?
    (A) IV medication may be administered, but space at longer than standard intervals.
    (B) Withhold medications until the core temperature is 90°F.
    (C) IV medications may be administered at regular intervals.
    (D) Lidocaine and procainamide will increase fibrillation threshold.

58. Care during transportation for this patient should include all of the following except
    (A) avoiding rough handling due to cardiac irritability.
    (B) protection against further heat loss.
    (C) transporting in a horizontal position.
    (D) withholding further ACLS treatment until core temperature is >90°F.

---

59. All of the following are signs and symptoms of organophosphate poisoning except

    (A) salivation.
    (B) lacrimation.
    (C) urination.
    (D) tachycardia.

60. Which of the following is true regarding frostbite?
    (A) Superficial frostbite involves freezing of the epidermal and subcutaneous tissue.
    (B) Do not thaw frozen flesh if there is any possibility of refreezing.
    (C) Massage the frozen area lightly.
    (D) Do not elevate frozen extremities.

61. Physical assessment findings, signs, or symptoms that support your suspicion that a patient is under the influence of alcohol or drugs include
    1. chest pain and dysrhythmias
    2. confusion and polyuria
    3. dilated pupils and anxiety
    4. constricted pupils and respiratory depression
    (A) 1 and 2.
    (B) 2 and 3.
    (C) 2, 3, and 4.
    (D) All of the above.

Questions 62–64 are based on the following scenario:
You are called to the scene of a 46-year-old female who is unresponsive. Her husband states that he just came home from work and found her on the floor in the bathroom. She has a history of depression for which she receives outpatient treatment. There are acetaminophen and Valium found strewn around the room. Your best assessment of the situation speculates that the patient may have ingested one hundred 500 mg acetaminophen and ten 5 mg Valium. You notice the smell of alcohol on the patient.

62. What would be considered the worst outcome of an acetaminophen overdose?
   (A) internal bleeding.
   (B) nausea and vomiting.
   (C) liver failure and death.
   (D) cardiac dysrhythmias.

63. Her vital signs are BP 72/40, pulse 128, respirations 6. What is most likely the primary cause of the hypotension, tachycardia, and respiratory depression?
   (A) Alcohol intoxication
   (B) Acetaminophen ingestion
   (C) Valium ingestion
   (D) Hypoglycemia

64. Which statement is true regarding the administration of Narcan to this patient?
   (A) Narcan will not reverse the effects of Valium.
   (B) Narcan should be administered to this patient since it is uncertain if any opiates were ingested.
   (C) A proper dose range is 1–2 mg IVP.
   (D) All of the above.

---

65. Which of the following statements about delirium tremens is false?
   (A) DTs can occur from either an abrupt discontinuation or ingestion of alcohol after prolonged use.
   (B) Withdrawal symptoms usually occur after one week of abstinence.
   (C) DTs are characterized by a decreased level of consciousness and hallucinations.
   (D) There is significant mortality associated with DTs.

66. You are called to a local restaurant for a patient exhibiting bizarre behaviors and shouting obscenities. He is pale, diaphoretic, and denies any past medical problems. Which of the following interventions would be most appropriate?
    (A) Place patient in 4 point restraints.
    (B) Administer Valium 10 mg as a sedative.
    (C) Rapid sequence intubation and hyperventilate to decrease intracranial pressure.
    (D) Fingerstick to check blood glucose.

67. You are called to assist a 25-year-old known Type I diabetic patient who is complaining of abdominal pain, vomiting, and lethargy. His glucometer reading is 510. The highest treatment priority for this patient is to
    (A) reverse alkalosis by hyperventilation.
    (B) administer patient's next scheduled dose of insulin intravenously.
    (C) correct fluid volume deficit.
    (D) administer morphine to provide for pain management.

68. A patient's glucometer reads 66. You may encounter all of the following symptoms of hypoglycemia except
    (A) altered mental status.
    (B) hot, dry skin.
    (C) bizarre behavior.
    (D) hunger.

Questions 69 and 70 are based on the following scenario:
A 42-year-old male presents with severe pain in the left flank area with no history or signs of trauma. The patient has excruciating colicky pain with intermittent vomiting.

69. What problem would you suspect as the cause of the patient's discomfort?
    (A) Abdominal aortic aneurysm
    (B) Appendicitis
    (C) Gallbladder attack
    (D) Renal calculi

70. Treatment for this patient would include
    (A) IV fluids and morphine.
    (B) a nasogastric tube to decompress the stomach.
    (C) NTG and aspirin.
    (D) PASG and 2 large-bore IVs wide open.

71. When ventilating a patient via an endotracheal tube, the amount of air flowing into the lungs will be reduced if
    (A) the patient is a young adult.
    (B) there is increased airway resistance.
    (C) the bronchi are dilated.
    (D) the chest expands easily with each ventilation.

72. Bradycardia and hypotension following an overaggressive dialysis treatment are MOST indicative of
    (A) hypovolemia.
    (B) hypokalemia.
    (C) hyperkalemia.
    (D) air embolism.

73. Which of the following is often a late finding in patients with respiratory distress?
    (A) Assuming an upright, tripod position
    (B) Restlessness and agitation
    (C) Cyanosis
    (D) Diaphoresis

Questions 74–79 are based on the following scenario:
You are called to attend to an 18-year-old male who is having a severe asthma attack. He is awake and alert but appears very tired. His vital signs are blood pressure 158/90, pulse 132, respiratory rate 32 and extremely labored.

74. Upon auscultation of his chest you note breath sounds heard only in the upper lobes with very little wheezing bilaterally. This is significant because it shows
    (A) bronchoconstriction with air trapping.
    (B) the lack of prominent wheezes, which rules out an asthma attack.
    (C) bronchodilation with adequate tidal volume.
    (D) the patient is not hypoxic.

75. His fatigue is significant in that it tells you
    (A) he is not in any danger of respiratory failure.
    (B) he is exchanging gases well in his lungs.
    (C) he is in danger of respiratory failure.
    (D) his condition is going to improve soon.

76. He is tachycardic at a rate of 132 beats per minute and has pale and diaphoretic skin. What is causing these signs?
    (A) Hypoxia
    (B) Suppression of the sympathetic nervous system
    (C) Release of epinephrine and norepinephrine
    (D) Both A and C are correct.

77. Why is he able to talk only in short, broken phrases?
    (A) His tachycardia is impairing perfusion.
    (B) He is in left ventricular failure.
    (C) His tidal volume is inadequate for him to speak in full sentences.
    (D) He is hypoxic.

78. Which intervention will assist in dilating his airways?
    (A) Supplemental oxygen via nonrebreather mask at 15 LPM
    (B) Administration of a nebulized beta-2 agonist
    (C) Allowing him to continue to sit upright
    (D) Starting an intravenous solution

79. What medication can be administered into the subcutaneous tissues to help alleviate his respiratory distress?
    (A) Benadryl 25 mg
    (B) epinephrine 1:10,000, 1 mg
    (C) Benadryl 5 mg
    (D) epinephrine 1:1,000, 0.3 mg

Questions 80–84 are based on the following scenario:
Your EMS team is dispatched to care for a 39-year-old female with difficulty breathing. She is awake and appears restless and apprehensive. She tells you she had sudden onset of shortness of breath and a "sense of doom" while typing on her computer keyboard. Her vital signs are: blood pressure 148/92; radial pulse is strong at 124 beats per minute; respiratory rate is 36 per minute and shallow. Her skin is pale, cool, and dry. She denies having chest pain or any health problems.

80. Your patient's pulse oximetry reading is 89% on room air. This indicates
    (A) that she is breathing too deeply.
    (B) that her breathing is within normal limits.
    (C) that she has hypoxemia.
    (D) that she has psychogenically induced hyperventilation syndrome.

81. What is significant about her apprehension and sense of doom?
    (A) It may indicate a threat to life.
    (B) It can safely be ignored at this time.
    (C) It is not related to her shortness of breath.
    (D) These problems can be easily controlled with diazepam (Valium).

82. During your interview, you find that the patient takes birth control pills and has had left calf tenderness for two days with no history of trauma to the area. This information leads you to suspect
(A) viral pneumonia.
(B) pulmonary edema.
(C) a panic attack.
(D) a pulmonary embolus.

83. You interpret her cardiac rhythm as

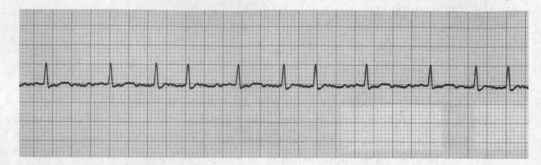

(A) junctional tachycardia.
(B) sinus tachycardia with premature atrial contractions (PACs).
(C) atrial fibrillation with a rapid ventricular response.
(D) super ventricular tachycardia.

84. Management of her condition would include all of the following except
(A) being on alert for cardiac arrest.
(B) administering nitroglycerin sublingually.
(C) monitoring the cardiac rhythm.
(D) establishing intravenous access.

---

85. A disease that results from the destruction of the walls of the alveoli and lessens the amount of surface area for gas exchange is termed

(A) emphysema.
(B) chronic bronchitis.
(C) asthma.
(D) pneumonia.

86. Patients with chronic obstructive pulmonary disease (COPD) often breathe through pursed lips to increase pressure in the lungs. This method of breathing helps in
(A) decreasing the blood carbon dioxide levels.
(B) preventing alveolar collapse.
(C) preventing the loss of elasticity in the lungs.
(D) reversing peripheral vasoconstriction.

87. In COPD, changes in the bronchioles that can result in significant air trapping include
    (A) inflammation.
    (B) bronchospasm.
    (C) increased mucus production.
    (D) all of the above are correct.

Questions 88–92 are based on the following scenario:

A 64-year-old male presents with increased dyspnea. He has a barrel chest, is thin, and is pink in color. Clubbing of the fingers is present. Wheezes and rhonchi are present bilaterally in all lobes, and pursed lip breathing is noted. Vital signs are: blood pressure 162/92; pulse 118 beats per minute; respiratory rate 22.

88. This patient's appearance suggests that he most likely is suffering from
    (A) pneumonia.
    (B) COPD.
    (C) asthma.
    (D) spontaneous pneumothorax.

89. The wheezes auscultated bilaterally indicate
    (A) narrowing of the airways.
    (B) partial obstruction by the tongue.
    (C) fluid in the smaller airways.
    (D) pleural inflammation.

90. The rhonchi auscultated bilaterally indicate
    (A) partial obstruction by the tongue.
    (B) fluid in the smaller airways.
    (C) excessive mucus in the larger airways.
    (D) a pleural friction rub.

91. The clubbing of the fingers is associated with
    (A) pulsus paradoxus.
    (B) respiratory disease.
    (C) an excess of red blood cells.
    (D) chronic dilation of the bronchioles.

92. The "pink" color of this patient's skin is a result of
    (A) an excess of circulating red blood cells.
    (B) high oxygen blood levels.
    (C) chronic dilation of the bronchioles.
    (D) wheezing.

Questions 93–95 are based on the following scenario:
A 19-year-old male is found breathing very rapidly. His roommate tells you he has been having a stressful time lately and recently lost his job. The patient is awake, alert, and very anxious. You note that he has spasms of his fingers and feet. Vital signs are blood pressure 130/78, pulse rate 116, respiratory rate 44 and regular. He takes no medications and has no past medical problems.

93. Hyperventilation resulting from pure anxiety leads to
    (A) respiratory acidosis.
    (B) respiratory alkalosis.
    (C) a decreasing blood pH.
    (D) hepatic failure.

94. Spasms of the hands and feet is termed
    (A) hypercalcemic contractions.
    (B) bronchospasm.
    (C) proximal extremity spasms.
    (D) carpopedal spasms.

95. In this situation, it is important to
    (A) withhold oxygen.
    (B) have the patient breathe into a paper bag as a rebreathing technique.
    (C) consider that he has a serious medical problem.
    (D) offer reassurance to him.

---

96. A medication that can assist in reversing bronchospasm is
    (A) albuterol.
    (B) nitroglycerin.
    (C) Benadryl.
    (D) both A and B.

97. Upper respiratory infections (URI) are more severe in which of the following patients?
    (A) Patients with asthma or COPD
    (B) Patients with HIV infection
    (C) Patients with mild hypertension
    (D) Both A and B

98. A skin rash, a metallic taste in the mouth, and explosive diarrhea are MOST indicative of
    (A) lead poisoning.
    (B) cyanide poisoning.
    (C) arsenic poisoning.
    (D) mercury poisoning.

Questions 99–101 are based on the following scenario:

You are called to attend to a 61-year-old female complaining of headache, vomiting, abdominal pain, and loss of coordination. She has recently been using a gas home-heating device to warm up her bedroom. Her sister lives next door and they always eat every meal together. The patient cannot get out of bed saying she is too tired. She appears to be sleeping now.

99. Upon assessing the patient, you note that she can speak clearly, slowly moves all extremities, and has a blood pressure of 164/86, pulse regular at 104, respiratory rate at 18 with normal effort. She has not eaten since last evening when she ate dinner with her sister. Her sister, however, feels fine. The patient's condition suggests
    (A) food poisoning.
    (B) carbon monoxide poisoning.
    (C) a cardiac disorder.
    (D) transient ischemic attack (TIA).

100. Her pulse oximetry is 99%. This can be misleading because
    (A) pulse oximetry is inaccurate in certain cases of poisoning.
    (B) the hemoglobin is fully saturated with oxygen.
    (C) the carbon dioxide blood level is dangerously low.
    (D) the carbon dioxide level is normal.

101. Which of the following is most important?
    (A) Provide high-flow oxygen
    (B) Apply a nasal cannula
    (C) Obtain a detailed history from the sister
    (D) Continue reassessment for acute CVA

102. A diagnostic device for measuring forced exhalation is a (an)
    (A) pulse oximeter
    (B) capnometer
    (C) peak flow meter
    (D) end-tidal CO_2 detector

103. Which device listed below would be most effective in determining if an endotracheal tube is placed in the stomach?
    (A) Pulse oximeter.
    (B) CPAP device.
    (C) Peak flow meter.
    (D) End-tidal CO_2 detector.

104. A peak flow value of 100 (liters/min) shows
    (A) normal value.
    (B) mild severity.
    (C) moderate severity.
    (D) severe respiratory compromise.

105. The process of gas exchange between the alveoli and the pulmonary capillary bed is termed
    (A) ventilation.
    (B) diffusion.
    (C) perfusion.
    (D) osmosis.

106. Side effects of albuterol (Proventil, Ventolin) administration include
    (A) hypotension and bradycardia.
    (B) pallor and sedation.
    (C) tachycardia and tremor.
    (D) respiratory depression.

107. Of the following choices, which is not a predisposing factor contributing to the development of pneumonia?
    (A) Alcoholism
    (B) Cigarette smoking
    (C) Extremes of age
    (D) Chest pain

108. A patient is anxious and has been breathing rapidly and deeply for the past 45 minutes. You can expect his blood carbon dioxide level to be
    (A) elevated.
    (B) decreased.
    (C) normal.
    (D) acidotic.

109. When the entire lobe of a lung is filled with infection and cellular debris, it is termed
    (A) pleuritic disease.
    (B) mild aspiration.
    (C) consolidation.
    (D) hemoptysis.

110. An antiinflammatory medication that can be used to treat asthma or chronic obstructive pulmonary disease (COPD) is
    (A) Proventil.
    (B) Alupent.
    (C) Solu-Medrol.
    (D) Benadryl.

111. Which medication and dosage is correct for a person with a long history of COPD and cardiac disease that presents with sudden onset of dyspnea who you believe is suffering acute pulmonary edema?
    (A) Nitroglycerin 4.0 mg
    (B) Furosemide (Lasix) 40 mg IV
    (C) Morphine sulfate 20 mg IV
    (D) Epinephrine (adrenalin) 1:1,000 0.3 SQ

112. A syndrome that develops as a complication of an illness such as multisystem trauma, severe sepsis, or toxic inhalation is termed
    (A) adult respiratory syndrome (ARDS).
    (B) pneumonia syndrome (PS).
    (C) chronic obstructive pulmonary disease (COPD).
    (D) congestive heart failure (CHF).

113. An expression of uncontrolled growth of abnormal lung cells is best termed
    (A) pulmonary disease.
    (B) chronic bronchitis.
    (C) lung cancer.
    (D) viral pneumonia.

114. A 49-year-old male with COPD is tired, confused, and in severe respiratory distress. His altered mental status is most likely caused by
    (A) carbon dioxide excretion.
    (B) hypoxia.
    (C) tachypnea.
    (D) Both A and B.

115. The MOST common and reliable sign of pit viper envenomation is
   (A) tachycardia within 30 seconds of the bite.
   (B) rapidly developing edema around the bite area.
   (C) patient anxiety and a slow, bounding pulse.
   (D) swelling of the tongue and marked hypertension.

116. Why is it important to limit the time for suctioning a patient's airway?
   (A) The blood carbon dioxide will decrease.
   (B) The blood oxygen level will decrease.
   (C) Bradycardia can develop.
   (D) Both B and C are correct.

117. You are called to attend to a patient who fell seven feet from a porch and landed on his head. He is unresponsive, has erratic respirations, and is bleeding from a head wound. Your first action to manage the airway would be
   (A) nasotracheal intubation.
   (B) head-tilt, chin-lift.
   (C) jaw thrust.
   (D) to initiate in-line traction with intubation.

118. A 58-year-old female has a history of smoking two packs of cigarettes per day. She suffers from frequent upper respiratory infections with a productive cough and expectorates white, thick phlegm. She most likely is suffering from
   (A) asthma.
   (B) congestive heart failure.
   (C) chronic bronchitis.
   (D) bronchiolitis.

119. Minute respiratory volume is best described as
   (A) the volume of air exhaled during the first minute of forced exhalation.
   (B) the volume of air moving through the alveoli in one minute.
   (C) a small amount of air being exchanged in the alveoli over one minute.
   (D) the amount of air moved in and out of the lungs during one minute.

120. The term orthopnea refers to
   (A) dyspnea while lying in the supine position.
   (B) shortness of breath while standing upright.
   (C) dyspnea while lying in the prone position.
   (D) shortness of breath while sitting upright in bed.

121. A 23-year-old healthy male who has been threatened by another person has a pulse rate of 146 and a respiratory rate of 32. These vital signs indicate that his
    (A) sympathetic nervous system is activated.
    (B) parasympathetic nervous system is activated.
    (C) sympathetic nervous system is blocked.
    (D) somatic nervous system is activated.

Questions 122–127 are based on the following scenario:

A 66-year-old female, is unable to get out of bed. She responds to verbal stimuli with clear speech, her smile is asymmetrical, she cannot move her left leg, and weakly moves her left arm. Her skin is warm but pale. Vital signs are: BP 162/88, pulse 110 beats per minute and irregular, respiratory rate 22 per minute with lung sounds clear bilaterally. A blood glucose reading is 130 mg/dl. The cardiac monitor shows a very irregular, narrow complex tachycardia with no identifiable P waves.

122. Damage to what body system is affecting movement of the left side of her body?
    (A) Cardiovascular system
    (B) Central nervous system
    (C) Pulmonary system
    (D) Endocrine system

123. The patient's asymmetrical smile is most likely a direct result of
    (A) damage to cranial nerve VII.
    (B) injury to the medulla oblongata.
    (C) damage to cranial nerve III.
    (D) cardiac disease.

124. Why was it important to obtain a blood glucose reading on this patient?
    (A) Blood glucose readings can help determine if the patient is an alcoholic.
    (B) Dextrose 50% in water can often reverse the effects of stroke.
    (C) Diabetics are less prone to stroke than healthy individuals.
    (D) Hypoglycemia can mimic stroke.

125. Her cardiac rhythm is
    (A) first-degree AV block.
    (B) atrial fibrillation.
    (C) sinus tachycardia.
    (D) second-degree AV block.

126. This cardiac rhythm makes her more prone to the development of
    (A) diabetes.
    (B) emboli.
    (C) brain tumors.
    (D) cardiogenic shock.

127. A family member states that she was fine one hour ago when he talked to her on the telephone. This is important information because
    (A) there is a six-hour window for treating occlusive strokes with thrombolytics.
    (B) it rules out a problem affecting her cerebral hemispheres.
    (C) it establishes a reference point for the onset of symptoms.
    (D) it clearly proves that she has an intracranial hemorrhage.

128. Stroke, or brain attack, can be compared to a heart attack in that
    (A) both have the same signs and symptoms.
    (B) in both cases, oxygen deprivation causes tissue damage.
    (C) thrombolytics can be beneficial in treating certain heart and brain attacks.
    (D) Both B and C are correct.

129. You are transporting a patient who is under the influence of methamphetamine. The patient, who is clearly anxious, has a BP 176/92, a pulse of 146, and respirations of 24. The patient suddenly becomes violent and begins thrashing around, trying to get off the stretcher. You should
    (A) assess his blood glucose level.
    (B) start an IV line and give him morphine.
    (C) administer a beta blocker and reassess.
    (D) administer intramuscular haloperidol.

Questions 130–133 are based on the following scenario:

A 30-year-old suddenly developed a two- to three-minute grand mal seizure. On scene you find an unconscious and unresponsive patient with the following vital signs: BP 178/100, pulse 50 and regular, respiratory rate 32 and irregular. He has no history of substance abuse but has complained of headaches for the past two weeks. His blood glucose registers 110.

130. You suspect that his problem is most likely the result of
    (A) hypoglycemia.
    (B) a structural lesion.
    (C) hyperglycemia.
    (D) atrial fibrillation.

131. Two minutes after the insertion of an oropharyngeal airway, applying high-flow oxygen, and assisting his ventilations with a bag-valve mask, the patient's pulse oximetry reading is 90%. His skin is pale and moist. It is important to consider
    (A) starting two large-bore IVs.
    (B) immediate transport to a hospital.
    (C) immediate endotracheal intubation.
    (D) immediate placement of a nasopharyngeal airway.

132. It is important to avoid excessive hyperventilation because it can
    (A) increase the blood $PaCO_2$ to dangerously high levels.
    (B) decrease the blood $PaCO_2$ to dangerously low levels.
    (C) cause jugular vein distention.
    (D) vasodilate the brain's vasculature.

133. The patient is now exhibiting decorticate posturing to painful stimuli. These are signs that indicate
    (A) decreased peripheral perfusion.
    (B) a lesion of the spinal cord.
    (C) decreased $PaCO_2$ blood levels.
    (D) a lesion at or above the upper brainstem.

Questions 134 and 135 are based on the following scenario:

You are called to attend to a 51-year-old male who fell in his living room. His wife states that he has been very depressed and has not eaten or drunk anything for the past 24 hours. You notice that the patient has a stonelike face, muscular rigidity, and is exhibiting "pill-rolling" movements.

134. These are all signs of
    (A) multiple sclerosis.
    (B) Bell's palsy.
    (C) Parkinson's disease.
    (D) vertebral disc disease.

135. In managing this patient, it is important to
    (A) start an intravenous line.
    (B) determine a blood glucose level.
    (C) apply a cardiac monitor.
    (D) All of the above are correct.

136. In differentiating between syncope and a grand mal seizure, you know that syncope
    (A) often begins in a standing position.
    (B) presents with jerking motions during unconsciousness.
    (C) causes the patient to remain drowsy following the event.
    (D) is often preceded by an aura.

Questions 137 and 138 are based on the following scenario:

A 27-year-old patient is complaining of persistent headache, fatigue, and pain upon flexion of his neck. He has had a chronic fever of 100°F for the past two days.

137. His complaints lead you to suspect
    (A) Reye's syndrome.
    (B) meningitis.
    (C) transient ischemic attack.
    (D) a mental disorder.

138. In treating this patient, you would
    (A) wear gloves and place a mask on yourself and the patient.
    (B) wear gloves only.
    (C) transport the patient to a hospital that can administer thrombolytics.
    (D) arrange for a psychiatric consult to meet you at the hospital.

---

139. A seizure characterized by a rapid mood change or auras that include unusual smells, tastes, or sounds is termed
    (A) simple partial seizure disorder.
    (B) petit mal seizure disorder.
    (C) pseudoseizure disorder.
    (D) complex partial seizure disorder.

140. You are having lunch with your nephew Josh and his friend Sam. You notice that Sam appears to have periods of inattentiveness and daydreaming. During these spells, his eyelids flutter and he appears to be unaware of his surroundings. You ask Josh if he has ever noticed this before. Josh says he has been "goofing around" like this for a week now. These signs indicate Sam may have
    (A) simple partial seizure disorder.
    (B) petit mal seizure disorder.
    (C) pseudoseizure disorder.
    (D) complex partial seizure disorder.

Questions 141–144 are based on the following scenario:

Your EMS team is called to attend to a patient in her mid-thirties who is having a generalized motor seizure. Bystanders inform you that she has been seizing continually for the past 10 minutes. You note that the patient is shaking violently, is diaphoretic, and slightly cyanotic.

141. This prolonged seizure is specifically termed
    (A) petit mal seizure disorder.
    (B) grand mal seizure disorder.
    (C) complex seizure disorder.
    (D) status epilepticus.

142. The most valuable early intervention is to
    (A) force an oropharyngeal airway between the teeth.
    (B) start an IV of crystalloid solution.
    (C) use bag-valve mask assistance with 100% oxygen.
    (D) give dextrose 50% and water IVP.

143. An IV is started and blood glucose reading is 120 mg/dl. A medication and correct dose range that you could administer to her is
    (A) Valium (diazepam) 5–10 mg IVP.
    (B) dextrose 50% in water 5–10 grams.
    (C) Valium (diazepam) 5–10 mcg IVP.
    (D) Versed (midazolam) 10–25 mg IVP.

144. Administration of the medication terminated her seizure activity. Now you should be alert for which of the following side effects?
    (A) Respiratory depression
    (B) Hyperglycemia
    (C) Hypertension
    (D) Fever

---

145. Your EMS unit is called to attend to a 79-year-old female who experienced an abrupt onset of facial drooping, dysphasia, and marked hemiparesis. Upon examination, she is now alert and oriented, speech clear, and moves all extremities well. Vital signs are normal. Your assessment findings lead you to suspect
    (A) stroke.
    (B) transient ischemic attack.
    (C) Alzheimer's disease.
    (D) amyotrophic lateral sclerosis.

146. Intracranial hemorrhage can cause vital sign changes characterized by an increasing systolic blood pressure and widening pulse pressure, bradycardia, and irregular respiratory rate. These changes are collectively termed
    (A) Cheyne-Stokes respiration.
    (B) Cushing's reflex.
    (C) Wernicke's syndrome.
    (D) hypertensive crisis.

147. One area that the Glasgow Coma Scale measures is
    (A) pupillary response and size.
    (B) respiratory rate.
    (C) heart rate.
    (D) motor response.

148. _____ injuries are tissue disruptions that occur directly at the point of impact.
    (A) Concussion
    (B) Contrecoup
    (C) Coup
    (D) Epidural

149. You have a patient with metastatic brain cancer. He opens his eyes to pain, and answers questions with incomprehensible sounds. When you start an IV in his left arm, he withdraws from the IV needle piercing the skin. You would calculate his Glasgow Coma Scale to be
    (A) 9.
    (B) 11.
    (C) 7.
    (D) 4.

150. Which of the following are signs/symptoms of an acute cerebral vascular accident?
    (A) Slurring of the speech
    (B) Facial droop
    (C) Drooling
    (D) Weak motor response on the affected side

ANSWERS AND ANSWER EXPLANATIONS

1. **(C)** With a presentation of confusion and diaphoresis, you should be thinking hypoglycemia. Of the choices listed, establishing an IV and obtaining a blood sample for a blood glucose test is the best answer. Choices (A) and (B) may need to be further evaluated, especially if the blood glucose test is within normal limits. (D) is not correct because you were not given enough information in the scenario to determine a cardiac origin.

2. **(D)** Morbidly obese patients in respiratory distress should be sat up or placed on their side. When a morbidly obese patient is supine, his/her own body weight can often impair the mechanics of respiration. This is known as Pickwickian syndrome.

3. **(A)** Polydipsia (excessive thirst), polyuria (excessive urination), and polyphagia (excessive hunger) are just a few symptoms of untreated diabetes mellitus.

4. **(D)** When the body is not able to use glucose as a primary source of energy, the body starts to break down adipose (fat) tissue as a source of energy. This fat-based metabolism results in a rise of blood ketones, which can lead to ketoacidosis.

5. **(C)** You must be familiar with signs and symptoms of the most common endocrine disorders. Agitation, emotional changes, insomnia, heat intolerance, weight loss, and exophthalmos are all common in Graves' disease. Graves' disease is the result of thyrotoxicosis (excessive thyroid hormones).

6. **(A)** Thyroid storm is a true medical emergency that requires expedited transport to definitive care. Drug therapy that will block the effects of the toxic level of thyroid hormone is required. If you chose Adenocard or verapamil for your answer, this is incorrect because these medications are not indicated for sinus tachycardia and you simply do not have enough information in this scenario to warrant its use.

7. **(B)** Hypoglycemia is associated with Cushing's syndrome due to excessive cortisol levels.

8. **(A)** Long-term effects of hyperadrenalism lead to paper thin (almost transparent) skin that can be easily bruised or torn. The disease process also results in delayed healing, so great care with venipuncture is required. (B) is incorrect because IV therapy is *not* contraindicated. (C) is incorrect because you should never make an assumption about a patient's blood glucose level.

9. **(A)** Hyperadrenalism is associated with high incidents of atherosclerosis, hypertension, and diabetes, which are all risk factors for stroke.

10. **(C)** Presentation of adrenal insufficiency (Addisonian crisis) may include cardiovascular collapse, hypotension, and hypoglycemia. These serious signs/symptoms are attributed to major disturbances in the water and electrolyte balance within the body.

11. **(B)** A delayed hypersensitivity reaction may occur several hours or even days after exposure. Common causes are medications and chemicals. A patient may very well present with the signs/symptoms of allergic reaction several days after starting a new medication.

12. **(B)** The teacher is experiencing a severe allergic (anaphylactic) reaction as evidenced by chest tightness, dyspnea, and inability to talk in complete sentences within five minutes of exposure.

13. **(C)** Because this patient is demonstrating pending cardiovascular and respiratory collapse, the administration of intravenous epinephrine is indicated. The correct dose range is 3 to 5 ml of 1:10,000 solution IV.

14. **(C)** The normal dose range of Benadryl is 25 to 50 mg. The online medical control order to administer such a large dose of Benadryl should be questioned.

15. **(C)** Melena is dark, tarry, foul-smelling stool that indicates the presence of partially digested blood.

16. **(C)** A patient who is unconscious and unresponsive with deep gasping respirations of eight per minute and inspiratory stridor requires assisted ventilations and endotracheal intubation. With the possibility of c-spine injury, proper precautions must be taken. **(D)** is incorrect because a rate of 24 ventilations per minute is too fast. **(A)** is incorrect because the respiratory rate is too slow to apply a nonrebreather mask. **(B)** is not a better answer than **(C)**.

17. **(C)** Based on the presence of bee stings, and the absence of obvious chest trauma causing the respiratory distress, you should suspect severe bronchial constriction secondary to anaphylactic reaction.

18. **(D)** Epinephrine 1:1,000 solution 0.3–0.5 mg SQ.

19. **(B)** Raised areas or wheals on the skin associated with allergic reaction and histamine release are known as urticaria (hives).

20. **(D)** The standard adult dose of subcutaneous epinephrine in the treatment of allergic reaction is 0.3–0.5 mg of 1:1,000 solution.

21. **(B)** Somatic pain is a sharp type of pain that travels along a definitive neural route. Visceral pain **(D)** is dull, poorly localized pain that originates in the walls of the hollow organs. Referred pain **(C)** is pain that originates in a region other than where it is felt. Peritonitis **(A)** is inflammation of the peritoneum.

22. **(D)** Visceral pain is dull, poorly localized pain that originates in the walls of the hollow organs. Somatic pain **(B)** is a sharp type of pain that travels along a definitive neural route. Referred pain **(C)** is pain that originates in a region other than where it is felt. Peritonitis **(A)** is inflammation of the peritoneum.

23. **(C)** Referred pain is pain that originates in a region other than where it is felt. Somatic pain **(B)** is a sharp type of pain that travels along a definitive neural route. Visceral pain **(D)** is dull, poorly localized pain that originates in the walls of the hollow organs. Peritonitis **(A)** is inflammation of the peritoneum.

24. **(C)** The correct assessment order of the abdomen is inspect, auscultate, palpate, percuss. Inspection is the obvious first step since you are going to look before you do anything. Auscultation may not provide much useful information but if you are going to auscultate, it must be performed before palpation. Palpation is the third step. You can gain a lot of information through palpation. Percussion (if performed) is the last assessment step.

25. **(A)** Ecchymosis in the periumbilical area in known as Cullen's sign. Grey-Turner's sign **(B)** is ecchymosis in the flank area. Both may indicate intraabdominal hemorrhage. Mallory-Weiss sign **(D)** is associated with an esophageal tear or laceration that results from excessive vomiting. Peritonitis **(C)** is inflammation of the peritoneum.

26. **(B)** The presence of Cullen's sign may indicate intraabdominal hemorrhage.

27. **(B)** An esophageal tear or laceration that results from excessive vomiting is known as a Mallory-Weiss tear. While you may suspect this type of injury, it is difficult to be 100% certain. Do not rule out more serious causes of upper GI bleeding.

28. **(B)** A subconjunctival hemorrhage involves rupture of small blood vessels in the subconjunctival space resulting in the "white" of the eye becoming blood red. This may occur after a strong sneeze or excessive vomiting. While it looks dramatic, this type of hemorrhage usually clears without intervention and rarely causes any residual problems.

29. **(A)** The usual dose range of Phenergan is 12.5 to 25 mg. It can be administered slow IVP or by deep IM injection. SQ administration is not indicated.

30. **(D)** Ecchymosis in the flank area associated with intraabdominal hemorrhage is known as Grey-Turner's sign. Ecchymosis in the periumbilical area in known as Cullen's sign **(B)**. Mallory-Weiss sign **(C)** is associated with an esophageal tear or laceration that results from excessive vomiting. Peritonitis **(A)** is inflammation of the peritoneum.

31. **(B)** The patient's past medical history and presentation should lead you to the conclusion of ruptured esophageal varices. **(A)** is incorrect because a Mallory-Weiss tear is usually not associated with significant blood loss. **(C)** and **(D)** are incorrect. You do not have enough information in the scenario to determine this.

32. **(B)** This patient is experiencing shock as evidenced by his elevated pulse rate (144), evidence of vasoconstriction (pale moist skin), and his ability to maintain his blood pressure.

33. **(B)** As always, the airway is your priority. You must protect the airway and prevent aspiration of emesis. Supplemental oxygen, establishing intravenous access, and treating this patient for shock are required. **(A)** and **(C)** are incorrect because Phenergan potentiates the effects of alcohol. **(D)** is incorrect because this patient needs supplemental oxygen and transport to an acute care hospital.

34. **(D)** Choice **(D)** is "Both **(B)** and **(C)** are correct." His vital signs indicate decompensated shock and rapid transport is necessary. While it is true alcohol is a CNS depressant and can alter mental status, you cannot assume this is the cause of his change in mental status since decompensated shock is present; therefore **(A)** is incorrect.

35. **(B)** 1.5–2.0 mg/kg is the initial dose of succinylcholine.

36. **(C)** 1.5–2.0 mg/kg is the initial dose of succinylcholine. A 186-pound (85-kg) patient would receive 127–170 mg of medication.

37. **(B)** Crohn's disease is an idiopathic inflammatory bowel disorder involving the small intestine.

38. **(D)** Diverticulitis is small outpouchings of mucosal and submucosal tissue that push through the outermost layer of the intestine.

39. **(B)** McBurney's point is a common site of pain from appendicitis and is located one to two inches above the anterior iliac crest in a direct line with the umbilicus.

40. **(A)** Rebound tenderness is pain on release of the examiner's hand, allowing the patient's abdominal wall to return to its normal position and is usually associated with peritoneal irritation. This assessment finding can be present in other abdominal conditions and is not specific to appendicitis.

41. **(B)** Pain and discomfort to the body can activate the sympathetic nervous system.

42. **(B)** Murphy's sign is pain caused when an inflamed gallbladder is palpated by pressing under the right costal margin. McBurney's point **(A)** is a common site of pain from appendicitis located one to two inches above the anterior iliac crest in a direct line with the umbilicus. Grey-Turner's sign **(C)** is ecchymosis in the flank area. Cullen's sign **(D)** is ecchymosis in the peri-umbilical area.

43. **(C)** All of the information presented in this scenario should have led you to the conclusion of cholecystitis (inflammation of the gallbladder).

44. **(B)** Demerol 25–50 mg IV is titrated for pain relief. **(A)** is incorrect, as morphine is contraindicated because it is believed to cause spasm of the cystic duct in the gallbladder. **(C)** and **(D)** are incorrect because the dosages listed are wrong. Note: While there might be concern about use of pain medication in "undiagnosed" abdominal pain or the administration of pain medication may mask symptoms and make in-hospital assessment more difficult, the use of Demerol is not contraindicated in cholecystitis.

45. **(B)** His history of alcoholism and presentation should lead you to suspect severe pancreatitis. Eighty percent of all cases of pancreatitis are associated with alcoholism.

46. **(C)** His BP of 86/42 and pulse of 138 lead you to believe a shock state is present. His temperature of 104.2°F may indicate sepsis. Severe pancreatitis is associated with septic shock, and when present it has a high mortality rate. **(A)** is incorrect because this scenario did not give you enough information to conclude that excessive vomiting caused hypovolemia. **(B)** is incorrect because these vital signs indicate shock and not a normal response to an infection.

47. **(A)** The inability to urinate is a true medical emergency because a full, distended bladder is extremely painful for the patient. Definitive care usually requires insertion of a urethral catheter, which is not common in the pre-hospital setting. EMS treatment is primarily supportive. **(C)** is incorrect because Demerol may cause urethral constriction and further complicate the problem. **(B)** is incorrect, the patient should be transported to the hospital by ambulance.

48. **(C)** Heat cramps are acute painful spasms of the voluntary muscles following strenuous activities in a hot environment.

49. **(A)** Treatment for heat cramps include removing the patient from the hot environment and administration of oral saline solution or sport drinks for hydration. If oral fluids cannot be administered because of nausea, an IV line of normal saline may be needed. **(C)** and **(B)** are incorrect because rapid cooling is indicated for heatstroke *not* heat cramps and two large-bore IVs are not indicated.

50. **(B)** Profuse sweating with *cool* and clammy skin, tachycardia, rapid shallow respiration, and a body temperature over 100°F indicates heat exhaustion.

51. **(D)** Treatment for heat exhaustion includes removal of clothing **(A)**, removal of the patient from the hot environment **(C)**, establishing an IV of normal saline **(B)**, and oral hydration if the patient is able to take fluids. The administration of salt tablets is *not* indicated because they are not readily absorbed through the stomach and can lead to hypernatremia.

52. **(A)** This patient has progressed from heat exhaustion to heatstroke as indicated by severe apprehension, hypotension, hot skin, and the cessation of sweating. Treatment for heatstroke includes removal of clothing, removal of the patient from the hot environment, establishing large-bore IVs of normal saline to run wide open, and rapid active cooling. One method of rapid active cooling is covering the patient in a sheet that has been soaked in *tepid* water. Using ice or cold water may cause a reflex hypothermia and cause the patient to shiver, which will raise the body temperature again.

53. **(C)** This choice is incorrect because overcooling of a heatstroke patient will produce a reflex hypothermia and cause the patient to shiver, which will raise the body temperature again. All of the other statements are true regarding over-cooling of a heatstroke patient.

54. **(D)** Hypothermia can result from an increase in heat loss, a decrease in heat production, or a combination of these two factors.

55. **(A)** CPR is indicated even if signs of death are present. Hypothermic patients cannot be presumed dead until a core body temperature of 94–95°F has been achieved and resuscitation efforts are still unsuccessful.

56. **(B)** Immediate defibrillation is required for this patient.

57. **(A)** IV medication may be administered, but spaced at longer than standard intervals, therefore **(C)** is incorrect. Drug metabolism is reduced so administered medication such as epinephrine and lidocaine may accumulate to toxic

levels. In addition, administered drugs may remain in the peripheral circulation. When the patient is rewarmed and peripheral circulation resumes, a large toxic bolus of medication may be delivered to the central circulation. **(D)** is incorrect because lidocaine and procainamide will actually lower fibrillation threshold in a severely hypothermic patient. **(B)** is incorrect because medications should be withheld when the core temperature is below 86°F.

58. **(D)** If the hypothermic cardiac arrest patient fails to respond to initial defibrillation attempts and drug therapy, subsequent ACLS care should be held until the core temperature is 86°F. **(D)** is incorrect because it states "90°F." **(A)**, **(B)**, and **(C)** are all true.

59. **(D)** SLUDGE is a helpful mnemonic to remember signs of poisoning— S = salivation, L = lacrimation, U = urination, D = defecation, G = GI upset, E = emesis. Other symptoms of organophosphate poisoning include bronchoconstriction, bradycardia, anxiety, and visual disturbances.

60. **(B)** A golden rule for the treatment of frozen flesh is to never thaw it if there is any possibility of refreezing. **(A)** is incorrect because deep frostbite involves freezing of the epidermal and subcutaneous tissue. **(C)** is incorrect because massaging frozen flesh may further damage the tissue

61. **(D)** While I'm not a fan of multiple-multiple guess questions such as this one, there is a possibility you may see this type of question format on a certification exam. The correct answer is All of the above. Chest pain and dysrhythmias are a typical sign/symptom of cocaine abuse. Confusion and polyuria represent alcohol use. Dilated pupils and anxiety represent evidence of hallucinogens. Constricted pupils and respiratory depression are the result of opiates.

62. **(C)** This patient may have ingested 50,000 mg of acetaminophen. A dose of 150 mg/kg of acetaminophen is considered toxic. Unless this patient weighed approximately 334 kg (734 lb) this is likely to be a toxic dose. Severe acetaminophen toxicity will often result in death within three to six days due to acute liver failure.

63. **(C)** Side effects of Valium or benzodiazepine ingestion include hypotension, respiratory depression, drowsiness, headache, blurred vision, nausea, and vomiting. Tachycardia is a compensatory mechanism of the body in response to the hypotension.

64. **(D)** Narcan is primarily used for complete or partial reversal of opiates. Valium is a benzodiazepine; therefore, Narcan will not reverse its effects. Romazicon is used to reverse effects of benzodiazepines. The administration of Narcan to this patient would not be unreasonable since it is unclear if the patient ingested opiates. A normal dose range of Narcan is 1–2 mg.

65. **(B)** This is false because DTs can occur several hours after sudden abstinence from alcohol and can last up to seven days.

66. **(D)** A glucose fingerstick is a quick tool to rule out hypoglycemia, which could be the cause of this patient's behavior. Any patient with an altered level of consciousness should be tested for hypoglycemia.

67. **(C)** This patient has diabetic ketoacidosis and is likely to be profoundly dehydrated because excess glucose acts as an osmotic diuretic. Fluid replacement with normal saline should be started immediately.

68. **(B)** The signs and symptoms of hypoglycemia are many and varied. Altered mental state including irritability, bizarre behavior, or agitation is often the most important and early indicator of a problem. Other signs/symptoms may include diaphoresis, tachycardia, weakness, and headache. Coma may be present in severe cases.

69. **(D)** Sudden onset of flank pain, excruciating colicky pain, and vomiting are considered classic signs and symptoms of renal calculi (kidney stones).

70. **(A)** Prehospital care should be focused on comfort and support. Give nothing by mouth and establish an IV line for medication administration. An antiemetic may be indicated, and pain management is important. Note: While there may be concern about the use of pain medication in "undiagnosed" abdominal pain or that administration of pain medication may mask symptoms and make in-hospital assessment more difficult, the use of morphine is not contraindicated in renal calculi.

71. **(B)** Airway resistance resulting from edema, bronchoconstriction, or increased mucus production can cause increased airway resistance, resulting in a decrease in the amount of air flowing into the lungs.

72. **(B)** Overaggressive dialysis treatment can lead to a reduction in potassium (hypokalemia). This is likely to be seen immediately after dialysis treatment.

73. **(C)** Cyanosis is a late finding and may not be present even when the patient is severely hypoxic.

74. **(A)** This assessment finding indicates that there is bronchoconstriction and air trapping. This serious condition results in decreased air exchange in the lungs and can lead to profound hypoxia.

75. **(C)** Fatigue in this situation indicates that the patient is becoming tired. This is an ominous sign of pending respiratory failure and the development of respiratory arrest.

76. **(D)** Both hypoxia and anxiety cause activation of the sympathetic nervous system and the release of epinephrine and norepinephrine, which causes diaphoresis, elevation of the heart rate (tachycardia), and peripheral vasoconstriction (pale skin).

77. **(C)** Because of the air trapping, he does not have enough air (tidal volume) available to speak.

78. **(B)** A nebulized beta-2 agonist (such as albuterol) delivered by mask or hand-held device using 5–10 LPM of oxygen can assist in bronchodilation.

79. **(D)** Subcutaneous epinephrine is an option to treat cases of severe asthma because of its beta-2 agonist properties.

80. **(C)** A pulse oximeter is used as an assessment tool. A patient with a pulse oximetry value of less than 90% with no apparent cause or past medical history is considered to be moderately hypoxic and needs high-flow oxygen administration.

81. **(A)** A patient who alerts you to his or her "sense of doom" should be taken very seriously. There are numerous reports of patients who have "sensed" a problem and later suffered a catastrophic event including a threat to life.

82. **(D)** A history of taking birth control pills combined with signs and symptoms that include a painful and inflamed lower extremity suggest deep vein thrombosis. This predisposes the patient to developing pulmonary embolus.

83. **(C)** This rhythm indicates atrial fibrillation with a rapid ventricular response.

84. **(B)** Nitroglycerin administration is inappropriate for this patient because the scenario did not give you enough information to warrant its use.

85. **(A)** Emphysema results from the destruction of the walls of the alveoli and lessens the amount of surface area for gas exchange. Chronic bronchitis **(B)** is the result of an increased number of mucus-secreting cells in the respiratory tree. Asthma **(C)** is a chronic inflammation disorder. Pneumonia **(D)** is an infection of the lung.

86. **(B)** Pursed-lip breathing technique helps maintain pressure within the airways (even during exhalation) to support bronchial walls that have been damaged as a result of disease.

87. **(D)** All of these pathologies impair the flow of air through the bronchial tree.

88. **(B)** A barrel chest, clubbing of the fingers, and dyspnea are all classic signs of COPD.

89. **(A)** Wheezes indicate narrowing of the airways. Edema and bronchoconstriction are examples of problems that can narrow the airway.

90. **(C)** Rhonchi are rattling sounds with a low pitch and "snoring quality" that is usually associated with excessive mucus or other material in the larger airways.

91. **(B)** Clubbing is a deformity produced by the growth of soft tissue about the fingers or toes. It is associated with chronic cardiac or respiratory disease.

92. **(A)** As part of the body's own compensatory mechanism, a chronic state of low blood oxygen levels will cause an increased production of red blood cells (polycythemia) that give the patient's skin a pink color.

93. **(B)** Hyperventilation can result in an excess elimination of carbon dioxide leading to respiratory alkalosis.

94. **(D)** Alkalosis decreases blood calcium levels, which leads to hypocalcemia. This results in cramping and spasms of the feet and hands.

95. **(C)** Since hyperventilation can mask a true medical emergency such as a pulmonary embolism, it is important to consider that this patient has a serious medical problem.

96. **(A)** Albuterol is a beta-2 agonist that dilates the bronchial tree.

97. **(D)** Patients with preexisting respiratory disease or who are immunocompromised are more prone to developing URI.

98. **(C)** Arsenic is the second leading cause of acute metal poisoning. Symptoms are a metallic taste in the mouth, explosive diarrhea, and severe abdominal pain.

99. **(B)** The home-heating device in the bedroom, the patient's signs and symptoms, and the fact that her sister is not sick should lead you to suspect carbon monoxide poisoning.

100. **(A)** Because carbon monoxide binds readily with the hemoglobin molecule, the pulse oximetry reading can read normal even though the patient may be hypoxic.

101. **(A)** Providing high flow oxygen is essential for a patient with carbon monoxide poisoning.

102. **(C)** The peak expiratory flow meter measures the amount of air a patient can forcefully exhale with one breath.

103. **(D)** This instrument measures the presence or absence of carbon dioxide in the sampled gas at the tip of the endotracheal tube. It can be used as an assessment tool to help determine proper endotracheal tube placement.

104. **(D)** A peak flow of 100 liters/min is very low; 400–650 liters/min is the normal range.

105. **(B)** Diffusion is the process of gas molecules moving across a cell membrane from a higher concentration of molecules to a lower concentration.

106. **(C)** Administration of albuterol can stimulate the sympathetic nervous system resulting in an increased heart rate and tremors.

107. **(D)** Chest pain may be a symptom of a problem but it is not a predisposing factor in itself. The very young and old, cigarette smokers, and alcoholism are all predisposing factors to the development of pneumonia.

108. **(B)** Rapid, deep breathing can result in excess elimination of carbon dioxide leading to respiratory alkalosis.

109. **(C)** The infection, debris, and fluid can fill up the lung creating consolidation.

110. **(C)** Solu-Medrol is a corticosteroid that can act as an antiinflammatory agent. It is commonly used in the treatment of COPD.

111. **(B)** Lasix is indicated for the treatment of acute pulmonary edema. **(A)** and **(C)** are incorrect because the dose is wrong. **(D)** is not indicated.

112. **(A)** ARDS is a form of pulmonary edema that occurs as a response to a wide variety of lung injury insults.

113. **(C)** Lung cancer is an excessive and uncontrolled growth of abnormal (cancerous) cells.

114. **(B)** Hypoxia can affect the brain at the cellular level resulting in a decreased mental status.

115. **(B)** Pit vipers include rattlesnakes, copperheads, and cottonmouths. Rapidly developing edema around the bite area can occur in as little as 15 minutes.

116. **(D)** Suctioning removes oxygen from the airway and can cause vagal stimulation resulting in bradycardia. Adults should not be suctioned for longer than 10–15 seconds. Pediatric patients should not be suctioned for longer than 5 seconds.

117. **(C)** From the choices listed, the modified jaw thrust is the easiest and safest method to manage the airway immediately.

118. **(C)** Years of exposure to toxic irritation (e.g., cigarettes) can result in an increase in the number of goblet cells in the bronchial system with an increased production of mucus.

119. **(D)** Minute volume is the amount of air moved in and out of the lungs in one minute.

120. **(A)** Dyspnea while lying supine best describes orthopnea.

121. **(A)** Sympathetic nervous system stimulation causes pupillary dilation and will increase the pulse and respiratory rates.

122. **(B)** An asymmetrical smile in conjunction with the inability to move her left leg and weakness of the left arm indicate injury to the patient's central nervous system (CNS).

123. **(A)** A patient's ability to smile, frown, lift eyebrows, and wrinkle the forehead is controlled by cranial nerve VII.

124. **(D)** Patients who are hypoglycemic can exhibit signs and symptoms similar to a stroke.

125. **(B)** Atrial fibrillation is an irregular, narrow complex rhythm with nondiscernible P waves.

126. **(B)** As the atria fibrillate, they also dilate. This allows for blood to stagnate in the atria and can lead to clot formation.

127. **(C)** Studies suggest that there is a three-hour window between the time of onset of symptoms and time of thrombolytic intervention for treatment to be effective. Establishing a reference point for the onset of symptoms is critical.

128. **(D)** Both heart attack and brain attack cause organ tissue damage due to the interruption of blood flow. Studies show that thrombolytic agents used to treat heart attack patients can be effective in treating occlusive strokes.

129. **(D)** A benzodiazepine such as haloperidol should be used to control anxiety caused by stimulant abuse. Chemical restraints are a widely accepted prehospital treatment.

130. **(B)** Structural lesions, such as brain tumors and intracerebral bleeds, can press on and destroy brain tissue. This can cause seizures and a number of other illnesses.

131. **(C)** A pulse oximetry reading of 90% in a person who is on high-flow oxygen indicates moderate hypoxia. Intubation should be considered.

132. **(B)** Excessive hyperventilation of a patient with increasing intracranial pressure can decrease the blood arterial carbon dioxide to dangerous levels.

133. **(D)** Decorticate posturing (flexion) indicates a lesion at or above the brainstem. Decerebrate posturing (extension), however, results from a lesion within the brainstem.

134. **(C)** Parkinson's disease is characterized by tremor, rigidity of muscles, bradykinesia, and impaired balance. It affects 500,000 Americans.

135. **(D)** Starting an intravenous line will allow access for medications if necessary, determining the blood glucose level will show if the altered mental status is due to hypoglycemia, and applying a cardiac monitor will determine if there is a rhythm disturbance.

136. **(A)** Syncope usually occurs when the person is in the standing position. It can begin with dizziness or feeling light-headed, or can occur without warning.

137. **(B)** Headache with fever, fatigue, and pain upon flexion of the neck are all suspicious signs and symptoms of meningitis.

138. **(A)** Universal precautions include use of gloves and a mask by the care provider as well as putting a mask on the patient, which significantly reduces the chance of exposure to the pathogen.

139. **(D)** A complex partial seizure disorder can present in many ways since they usually originate in the temporal lobe of the brain. They are usually of short duration and while patients experience a loss of contact with their surroundings, they do not lose motor tone.

140. **(B)** Petit mal, or absence, seizure is characterized by a brief loss of awareness for 10–30 seconds. This type of seizure occurs in childhood and usually disappears after 20 years of age.

141. **(D)** Status epilepticus is two or more generalized motor seizures occurring in succession and is a life-threatening emergency situation.

142. **(C)** Air exchange is poor during a generalized motor seizure. It is extremely important to protect the airway from obstruction and deliver 100% oxygen using a bag-valve mask for respiratory assistance.

143. **(A)** Valium (diazepam) is a sedative and anticonvulsant that depresses seizure activity in the brain. **(C)** and **(D)** are incorrect because the dose is wrong. **(B)** is not indicated with a blood glucose reading of 120 mg/dl.

144. **(A)** A side effect of Valium is respiratory depression.

145. **(B)** Since her signs and symptoms disappeared rapidly, and she has no neurological deficits, she most likely suffered a transient ischemic attack. TIA is considered a significant warning sign for the development of a stroke.

146. **(B)** Change in vital signs that are associated with increased intracranial pressure is termed Cushing's reflex.

147. **(D)** The Glasgow Coma Scale measures eye opening, and verbal response, and motor response.

148. **(C)** Coup injuries are tissue disruptions that occur directly at the point of impact. Contrecoup injuries **(B)** produce tissue damage away from (the opposite side) of the impact. Concussion **(A)** is a transient period of unconsciousness usually followed by a complete return of function. Epidural **(D)** is a location over or on the dura.

149. **(A)** You should always have a Glasgow Coma Scale chart available to reference in your EMS practice. Unfortunately, you may not have a chart to reference on a certification exam; therefore, you must be familiar with its contents. This patient has a GCS score of 9—eye opening = 2, verbal response = 3, motor response = 4.

150. **(A) (B) (C) (D)** All of these signs/symptoms may be present with an acute cerebrovascular accident. How long did you spend on this question? This is an example of a question with no obvious correct answer. You may experience this type of question on a certification exam. When this happens, keep cool and remember the advice on test taking that is found in Chapter One of this book.

Notes

Notes

Trauma

This chapter contains questions on assessment, recognition, and treatment of various traumatic injuries.

All ECG rhythm strips used in this chapter are six-second strips.

Answer Sheet
CHAPTER 5—TRAUMA

1 Ⓐ Ⓑ Ⓒ Ⓓ	21 Ⓐ Ⓑ Ⓒ Ⓓ	41 Ⓐ Ⓑ Ⓒ Ⓓ	61 Ⓐ Ⓑ Ⓒ Ⓓ
2 Ⓐ Ⓑ Ⓒ Ⓓ	22 Ⓐ Ⓑ Ⓒ Ⓓ	42 Ⓐ Ⓑ Ⓒ Ⓓ	62 Ⓐ Ⓑ Ⓒ Ⓓ
3 Ⓐ Ⓑ Ⓒ Ⓓ	23 Ⓐ Ⓑ Ⓒ Ⓓ	43 Ⓐ Ⓑ Ⓒ Ⓓ	63 Ⓐ Ⓑ Ⓒ Ⓓ
4 Ⓐ Ⓑ Ⓒ Ⓓ	24 Ⓐ Ⓑ Ⓒ Ⓓ	44 Ⓐ Ⓑ Ⓒ Ⓓ	64 Ⓐ Ⓑ Ⓒ Ⓓ
5 Ⓐ Ⓑ Ⓒ Ⓓ	25 Ⓐ Ⓑ Ⓒ Ⓓ	45 Ⓐ Ⓑ Ⓒ Ⓓ	65 Ⓐ Ⓑ Ⓒ Ⓓ
6 Ⓐ Ⓑ Ⓒ Ⓓ	26 Ⓐ Ⓑ Ⓒ Ⓓ	46 Ⓐ Ⓑ Ⓒ Ⓓ	66 Ⓐ Ⓑ Ⓒ Ⓓ
7 Ⓐ Ⓑ Ⓒ Ⓓ	27 Ⓐ Ⓑ Ⓒ Ⓓ	47 Ⓐ Ⓑ Ⓒ Ⓓ	67 Ⓐ Ⓑ Ⓒ Ⓓ
8 Ⓐ Ⓑ Ⓒ Ⓓ	28 Ⓐ Ⓑ Ⓒ Ⓓ	48 Ⓐ Ⓑ Ⓒ Ⓓ	68 Ⓐ Ⓑ Ⓒ Ⓓ
9 Ⓐ Ⓑ Ⓒ Ⓓ	29 Ⓐ Ⓑ Ⓒ Ⓓ	49 Ⓐ Ⓑ Ⓒ Ⓓ	69 Ⓐ Ⓑ Ⓒ Ⓓ
10 Ⓐ Ⓑ Ⓒ Ⓓ	30 Ⓐ Ⓑ Ⓒ Ⓓ	50 Ⓐ Ⓑ Ⓒ Ⓓ	70 Ⓐ Ⓑ Ⓒ Ⓓ
11 Ⓐ Ⓑ Ⓒ Ⓓ	31 Ⓐ Ⓑ Ⓒ Ⓓ	51 Ⓐ Ⓑ Ⓒ Ⓓ	71 Ⓐ Ⓑ Ⓒ Ⓓ
12 Ⓐ Ⓑ Ⓒ Ⓓ	32 Ⓐ Ⓑ Ⓒ Ⓓ	52 Ⓐ Ⓑ Ⓒ Ⓓ	72 Ⓐ Ⓑ Ⓒ Ⓓ
13 Ⓐ Ⓑ Ⓒ Ⓓ	33 Ⓐ Ⓑ Ⓒ Ⓓ	53 Ⓐ Ⓑ Ⓒ Ⓓ	73 Ⓐ Ⓑ Ⓒ Ⓓ
14 Ⓐ Ⓑ Ⓒ Ⓓ	34 Ⓐ Ⓑ Ⓒ Ⓓ	54 Ⓐ Ⓑ Ⓒ Ⓓ	74 Ⓐ Ⓑ Ⓒ Ⓓ
15 Ⓐ Ⓑ Ⓒ Ⓓ	35 Ⓐ Ⓑ Ⓒ Ⓓ	55 Ⓐ Ⓑ Ⓒ Ⓓ	75 Ⓐ Ⓑ Ⓒ Ⓓ
16 Ⓐ Ⓑ Ⓒ Ⓓ	36 Ⓐ Ⓑ Ⓒ Ⓓ	56 Ⓐ Ⓑ Ⓒ Ⓓ	76 Ⓐ Ⓑ Ⓒ Ⓓ
17 Ⓐ Ⓑ Ⓒ Ⓓ	37 Ⓐ Ⓑ Ⓒ Ⓓ	57 Ⓐ Ⓑ Ⓒ Ⓓ	77 Ⓐ Ⓑ Ⓒ Ⓓ
18 Ⓐ Ⓑ Ⓒ Ⓓ	38 Ⓐ Ⓑ Ⓒ Ⓓ	58 Ⓐ Ⓑ Ⓒ Ⓓ	78 Ⓐ Ⓑ Ⓒ Ⓓ
19 Ⓐ Ⓑ Ⓒ Ⓓ	39 Ⓐ Ⓑ Ⓒ Ⓓ	59 Ⓐ Ⓑ Ⓒ Ⓓ	79 Ⓐ Ⓑ Ⓒ Ⓓ
20 Ⓐ Ⓑ Ⓒ Ⓓ	40 Ⓐ Ⓑ Ⓒ Ⓓ	60 Ⓐ Ⓑ Ⓒ Ⓓ	80 Ⓐ Ⓑ Ⓒ Ⓓ

1. You are caring for a victim of a motor vehicle collision who has sustained multiple traumatic injuries. It has taken 15 minutes on the scene to secure your patient's airway, immobilize him on a backboard, and place him in the back of the ambulance. You are in a region in which the trauma care system consists of a Level I trauma center 50 minutes away and a Level III trauma center 10 minutes away. What is your choice of treatment facilities and why?
   (A) Level I trauma center because it is the only true center that is capable of handling trauma cases
   (B) Level I trauma center because you may be held liable if you take the patient to a facility of lesser capability.
   (C) Level III trauma center because it is capable of handling all types of specialty trauma
   (D) Level III trauma center because it will stabilize and transfer serious patients as needed as part of a trauma system

2. You are called to a scene of a motor vehicle collision (MVC). During your initial assessment, you find an unresponsive 32-year-old male with multiple contusions to his face and head. He has snoring respirations and a weak, thready peripheral pulse. Your first action would be
   (A) to control major bleeding.
   (B) rapid extrication.
   (C) to open the airway with a jaw thrust and immobilize the cervical spine.
   (D) endotracheal intubation and start two large-bore intravenous lines with normal saline and run at a "wide open" rate.

3. You perform a rapid trauma survey on an MBC victim and find him lethargic and very pale, with cool and clammy skin. He has contusions, crepitus, and diminished breath sounds on the right side of the chest. BP 74/50, pulse of 140 centrally, no peripheral pulse found at this time, and respirations 32 and shallow. What is the most likely cause of these findings?
   (A) Beck's triad
   (B) Hemopneumothorax
   (C) Cushing's syndrome
   (D) Ruptured liver

4. An initial assessment and rapid trauma survey should be completed in what length of time?
   (A) Five minutes
   (B) Ten minutes
   (C) Less than three minutes
   (D) Three to six minutes

5. You are called to the scene of a mass casualty incident where you are responsible for the triage transportation decisions. Which of the following patients would be the first to be transported to the local trauma center.
   (A) a 50-year-old man complaining of knee and ankle pain.
   (B) an 18-year-old female with a five-minute lapse of consciousness after being struck in the head
   (C) a 25-year-old female, eight months pregnant with partial thickness burns on her arms and legs covering 5% of her BSA
   (D) a 32-year-old male with a large piece of metal impaled in his left foot.

Questions 6–9 are based on the following scenario:

A 42-year-old male is the victim of a house fire. He has reddened and blistered areas over most of his anterior chest, abdomen, and anterior surfaces of both arms.

6. Using the rule of nines, estimate what percent of BSA he has burned.
   (A) 45%.
   (B) 36%.
   (C) 22.5%.
   (D) 27%.

7. Initial treatment for this burn patient would include which of the following?
   (A) Debridement of the blistered skin and antibiotic ointment
   (B) Covering the burn area with gauze and cooling with iced saline
   (C) Administering morphine and then cleaning the burn area with an iodine solution
   (D) Covering the burn area with dry bulky dressings and keeping the patient warm

8. Medical control has asked that you initiate fluid therapy enroute to the hospital. Which of the following statements regarding fluid resuscitation for this burn patient is true?
   (A) The Parkland Formula directs the fluid amount needed for the burn patient. It can be initiated only after a Foley catheter is in place so that accurate intake and output measurements can be monitored.
   (B) Two large-bore catheters are introduced and a bolus of 0.5 ml of normal saline (NS) for every kilogram of the patient's weight multiplied by the percentage of BSA is initiated.
   (C) Two large-bore IVs should run wide open for the length of the transport. Do not infuse more than 8,500 ml.
   (D) An IV is not attainable due to the location of the burns.

9. While transporting your burn patient to the burn center, you notice that his voice now sounds hoarse and he is making a "crowing" sound on inspiration. What is the most likely cause?
   (A) Screaming for help while standing inside the burning house
   (B) Fluid overload precipitating pulmonary edema
   (C) Allergic reaction to the by-products of the burning materials
   (D) Anxiety reaction to the traumatic event of being burned

10. A burn victim with suspected thermal or chemical airway burns needs close monitoring for signs of respiratory compromise. Appropriate management would include

    (A) immediate intubation using RSI upon all inhalation injuries.
    (B) using cool nebulized oxygen in a blow-by manner with a simple pocket mask to prevent further mucosal tissue damage.
    (C) providing high-flow oxygen by nonrebreather mask at 15 liters per minute once the airway has been secured.
    (D) suspecting cyanide toxicity and administering the sulfur-containing antidote.

11. Which one of the following statements is not true regarding electrical injuries?
    (A) Until the power is off, nobody should be allowed to approach the electrical burn patient.
    (B) The rescuer must be grounded to prevent electrical shock when treating a victim of a recent lightning strike.
    (C) Patients in cardiac arrest because of electrocution have a high survival rate if prehospital intervention is prompt.
    (D) Consider the use of 1 mEq/kg of sodium bicarbonate to prevent the complications of rhabdomyolyses.

12. Which of the following statements is true regarding chemical burns?
    (A) Always use antidotes or neutralizing agents.
    (B) Acid burns are typically more serious than alkali burns.
    (C) Both acids and alkalis cause burns by disrupting cell membranes and damaging tissues on contact.
    (D) Always approach a chemical spill from downwind.

Questions 13–15 are based on the following scenario:
You have arrived on scene where you find a 50-year-old male who has a large jagged laceration from a chain saw on his medial left upper thigh. Bright red blood is spurting from the wound. Your patient is alert, oriented, and anxious, with pale, diaphoretic skin.

13. What is the priority of care for this patient?
    (A) Two large-bore IVs wide open
    (B) Immobilize the c-spine and prepare to intubate
    (C) Tourniquet the upper right leg
    (D) Apply a pressure dressing while elevating the left leg

14. Your rapid trauma assessment reveals an isolated upper leg laceration that is seven inches in length and pumping bright red blood freely. His BP is 110/60, peripheral pulse 128, respiratory rate 24, and his GCS is 15. Several components of the circulatory system are essential for adequate profusion. Which of the following is not a component of the circulatory system?
    (A) Stroke volume and the Frank-Starlings mechanism
    (B) Positive end expiratory pressure
    (C) Preload and afterload
    (D) The pump, the fluid, and the container

15. Bleeding has been controlled and your patient is enroute to the trauma center. You instruct your partner to establish IV access and deliver fluid resuscitation. Pick the most appropriate treatment.
    (A) A bolus of normal saline or Ringer's lactate solution
    (B) Normal saline at "keep open" rate
    (C) Ringer's lactate at a "keep open" rate
    (D) Hold IV fluid infusion because your patient has a peripheral pulse

Questions 16–19 are based on the following scenario:

You are on duty at your EMS service when you are called to respond to a car that struck a light pole. As you arrive on scene you notice that power lines are down on top of the car. The driver is hanging halfway out of the driver's side window, unconscious, with slow, snoring-type respirations.

16. What is your first priority?
    (A) In-line stabilization of the c-spine and modified jaw thrust
    (B) Removing the wire from the top of the car and proceeding with caution
    (C) C-spine stabilization and oral pharyngeal airway with BVM ventilations
    (D) Calling the power company for assistance prior to starting patient care

17. After the patient is removed from the car, a rapid trauma survey shows a GCS of 9, BP 178/100, pulse 56, and respirations 34 and irregular. What is your differential diagnosis from this assessment?
    (A) Hypoglycemia
    (B) Hyperglycemia
    (C) Cushing's syndrome
    (D) CVA

18. To manage the airway of this patient appropriately you would
    (A) administer 100% O_2 by BVM at 30 breaths per minute.
    (B) use a nonrebreather mask on 10 liters of O_2.
    (C) use a nasal cannula on 10 liters of O_2.
    (D) intubate and hyperoxygenate with BVM at a rate of 24 breaths per minute

19. You have established two large-bore IVs of normal saline. Choose the appropriate rate.
    (A) Enough fluid to maintain stable vital signs
    (B) Both lines wide open
    (C) TKO
    (D) 500 cc bolus

20. Please choose the best clue for determining possible injuries that may be sustained in an MVC.
    (A) Length of skid marks
    (B) Debris at the scene
    (C) Patient symptoms
    (D) Mechanism of injury

21. Which of the following would you expect to cause the greatest cavitation?
    (A) a hunting knife
    (B) a bullet from a handgun
    (C) a bullet from a rifle
    (D) an arrow

Questions 22–24 are based on the following scenario:

You are called to the scene of a 60-year-old woman who fell down a flight of stairs. The patient is found to be alert and oriented, with warm, dry, and pink skin. She is complaining of a headache and upper back pain. Her vital signs are BP 90/62, pulse 60, and respiratory rate 20.

22. Which of the following would be your initial impression?
    (A) Neurogenic or distributive shock
    (B) No significant injury
    (C) The patient is taking beta-blockers
    (D) Mechanical shock

23. During your rapid trauma survey you find that the patient has no sensation below the border of the rib cage. This would suggest spinal pathology between which vertebral areas?
    (A) C1–C4
    (B) T4–T10
    (C) T10–S1
    (D) Below S1

24. You have started a large-bore IV normal saline on this patient. Choose the appropriate solution and rate.
    (A) Two large-bore IVs of normal saline wide open
    (B) Normal saline at a rate to maintain a systolic BP of 90
    (C) D5W TKO
    (D) 1,000 cc bolus of Ringer's lactate

Questions 25 and 26 are based on the following scenario:
You are called to the scene of a 22-year-old man who was playing in a softball tournament. He was hit in the eye with a hard-hit line-drive softball. According to his teammates he was knocked to the ground and had a brief loss of consciousness that lasted approximately seven seconds.

25. While assessing the injured eye you notice a collection of blood in front of the patient's pupil and iris. What is your differential diagnosis?
    (A) Raccoon's eye
    (B) Retinal detachment
    (C) Hyphema
    (D) Corneal laceration

26. How would you transport this patient to the hospital?
    (A) Recovery position
    (B) Sitting up at a 90 degree angle
    (C) Trendelenburg
    (D) Immobilized on a backboard with the head of backboard elevated

---

Questions 27 and 28 are based on the following scenario:

You are called to the scene of a patient who was involved in an altercation at the local pool hall. You find one victim in the back alley anxious and screaming for your assistance. You notice immediately that he has clammy skin and a dusky appearance. He has a respiratory rate of 40 and his breathing is shallow. He tells you that he has been hit multiple times in the chest, abdomen, and back with a pool stick by "two big guys." While assessing his chest you notice multiple contusions to the right side with diminished respirations on the right.

27. What would you suspect?
    (A) Cardiac tamponade
    (B) Hemothorax
    (C) Ruptured diaphragm
    (D) Pneumothorax

28. While enroute to the local trauma center with this patient, you notice that his level of consciousness has decreased and his color has not improved despite 100% O_2 by nonrebreather mask. He is becoming hypotensive and his pulse rate is 140. Respiratory rate remains at 40 and his breathing is still shallow. Ongoing assessment reveals distended neck veins and hyperresonant percussion on the right chest. Your next course of action would be
    (A) oropharyngeal intubation with RSI.
    (B) positive pressure ventilation with BVM.
    (C) needle decompression between the second and third intercostal space anterior chest.
    (D) to stabilize flail segment with a bulky dressing.

Questions 29 and 30 are based on the following scenario:
You are called to the scene of a stabbing. You find one victim lying supine on the ground in a large pool of blood with multiple lacerations to the abdomen. The scene is secure. Your initial assessment finds a patient responding only to pain with no peripheral pulse and respiratory rate of 8.

29. Priority care of this patient would be
    (A) MAST trousers and IV wide open.
    (B) BVM ventilations and moist saline dressings to the abdomen.
    (C) intubation and fluid resuscitation.
    (D) peritoneal lavage.

30. While transporting this patient to the hospital, a large section of bowel protrudes through one of the lacerations. Your management would be
    (A) to increase pressure in the abdominal compartment of MAST trousers.
    (B) to replace protruding bowel and apply a pressure dressing.
    (C) to make a note, no treatment necessary except to notify medical control.
    (D) to gently cover the area with moistened gauze and nonadherent material as a dressing.

Questions 31–33 are based on the following scenario:

You are called to the scene of an assault on a 75-year-old woman. She is unresponsive, with blood coming from the back of her head and multiple contusions and skin tears to her knees and arms. She has snoring respirations, a strong radial pulse of 60 beats per minute, and a moderate amount of bright red blood from a large laceration and hematoma in her occipital region.

31. What is your first priority?
    (A) Move the patient to an area for privacy.
    (B) Immediately stabilize the c-spine and open the airway.
    (C) Control bleeding with a pressure dressing to the head laceration.
    (D) Immediately load and go.

32. Why would this patient be more susceptible to severe head trauma?
    (A) A history of Alzheimer's disease
    (B) Dehydration
    (C) Pickwickian syndrome
    (D) Decreased size of the brain

33. After completing your rapid trauma assessment on your patient, you find a blood pressure of 96/54, heart rate of 50, and respiratory rate of 14 and regular. What is your priority of care?
    (A) Hyperventilation at a rate of 30 with 100% O_2
    (B) Two large-bore IVs at a wide-open rate
    (C) Careful fluid resuscitation
    (D) Atropine 0.5 mg IVP

Questions 34–36 are based on the following scenario:

You are called to the scene of a single-car MVC involving a 25-year-old female who is 30 weeks pregnant.

34. What normal physiological alterations take place during pregnancy that may affect your assessment of this patient?
    (A) Increased blood pressure and increased pulse
    (B) Increased blood pressure and decreased pulse
    (C) Decreased blood pressure and decreased pulse
    (D) Decreased blood pressure and increased pulse

35. You ascertain that this patient needs to be transported to the local trauma center for evaluation. What would be the best technique for the transport?
    (A) Properly secured to backboard and tilted to left side
    (B) Properly secured to backboard and tilted to right side
    (C) Position of comfort
    (D) Lithotomy position

36. During what month of gestation does the uterus rise out of the pelvic cavity and become more susceptible to blunt trauma?
    (A) Third month
    (B) Seventh month
    (C) Fifth month
    (D) Second month

Questions 37 and 38 are based on the following scenario:

A 5-year-old boy fell 10 feet from a jungle gym at school, hitting his head on the ground. Your initial evaluation reveals a child who is lethargic and does not respond appropriately to commands. His respirations are shallow at a rate of 40 with a rapid and weak radial pulse.

37. What is your first priority?
    (A) Splinting the deformed left leg
    (B) Wait for consent from the mother before giving definitive treatment
    (C) Application of c-collar and secure to backboard for immediate transport.
    (D) Rapid c-spine control and airway assistance with BVM and high-flow O_2

38. Which of the following is one of the most important indicators of potential CNS injury?
    (A) Ipsilateral pupil dilatation
    (B) History of loss of consciousness
    (C) Lethargy
    (D) Elevated heart rate.

39. Which of these should not be included in the documentation of baseline neurologic status?
    (A) Pulse oximetry
    (B) Response to sensory stimulation
    (C) Pupillary reaction
    (D) Motor function

40. Which of the following describes the most definitive treatment of a patient with a flail chest injury?
    (A) Position of comfort with O_2 per NRB mask
    (B) Intubation and positive pressure ventilation
    (C) Stabilization of the flail segment with a sandbag
    (D) Needle decompression

Questions 41 and 42 are based on the following scenario:

You arrive on scene to find a pickup truck that struck a utility pole head on. The patient is ambulatory on-scene. He is alert and oriented to person and place but slow to respond. You note the smell of alcohol on the patient as you speak with him.

41. You are sent to evaluate the damage to the truck. Which finding would lead you to believe the patient may have a life-threatening injury?
    (A) A deformed dashboard
    (B) A deformed steering wheel
    (C) The airbag did not deploy
    (D) Significant front end damage

42. It is important to remember that when dealing with an intoxicated patient, your assessment must be thorough because
    (A) alcohol increases pain tolerance.
    (B) alcohol decreases the patient's judgment.
    (C) alcohol is a CNS stimulant.
    (D) alcohol can mask signs and symptoms of injury.

43. One of the most common mechanisms of injury in the geriatric population is falls. Which statement is true regarding the force required to break a bone in a geriatric patient?
    (A) The same force is required as in other patients.
    (B) Less force is required than in other patients.
    (C) Slightly greater force is required than in other patients.
    (D) None of these statements are correct.

44. You arrive at the scene of a trench collapse. There are three trapped victims who are buried to the midchest. The rescue will take several hours because they will need to be dug out by hand. Crushing syndrome is a significant concern because crush injuries release toxins into the central circulation that can cause
    (A) alkalosis.
    (B) increased renal function.
    (C) cardiac dysrhythmias.
    (D) dyspnea.

45. Which medications would be given to a patient to combat the effects of crushing syndrome?
    (A) Narcan
    (B) Oxygen
    (C) Atropine
    (D) Sodium bicarbonate

46. You are caring for a 24-year-old male who wrecked his all-terrain vehicle. He states that his handlebar struck him in the stomach. He has bruising and tenderness in the abdomen and you suspect bowel rupture. This condition can lead to _____ and the development of serious complications.
    (A) peritonitis
    (B) diaphragm dysfunction
    (C) gastric distention
    (D) herniated bowel

Questions 47–50 are based on the following scenario:

You respond to a 25-year-old male involved in an industrial accident. Upon arrival, you see that your patient is trapped in a machine. He has suffered a partial amputation of the right leg just above the knee that is bleeding profusely.

47. Your first action is to
    (A) control bleeding.
    (B) stabilize the machinery.
    (C) do a rapid trauma assessment.
    (D) establish two large-bore IVs.

48. The patient remains trapped in the machine. He is awake, alert, and anxious. His blood pressure is 96/44, pulse 142, respiration 26. His skin is pale and moist. He is in what state of shock?
    (A) Decompensated
    (B) Compensated
    (C) Irreversible
    (D) Pneumatic

49. The patient has been freed from the machinery. Direct pressure and elevation do not stop the hemorrhage. The next step would be to apply
    (A) a tourniquet.
    (B) pressure at an arterial point proximal to the injury.
    (C) application of additional trauma dressings.
    (D) a vacuum splint.

50. Despite all efforts to control the bleeding, you are not successful. His pulse is now 52 and very weak. His respirations are 6 and labored. Blood pressure is 78/30. This shock state signifies
    (A) decompensated shock.
    (B) compensated shock.
    (C) irreversible shock.
    (D) pneumatic shock.

Questions 51–54 are based on the following scenario:

You are dispatched to a 77-year-old male patient who has fallen from a ladder while cleaning the gutters. He fell approximately 14 feet and struck the ground. He is awake and very anxious. He is having obvious trouble breathing. His pulse is 104, respirations 34, and blood pressure is 122/76. His wife tells you that he struck his back on the riding lawn mower as he fell.

51. In your assessment, you find crepitus and instability to the left rib cage. Lung sounds are present and equal. Closer assessment reveals paradoxical movement. You suspect a
    (A) tension pneumothorax.
    (B) massive hemothorax.
    (C) flail chest.
    (D) abdominal aneurysm.

52. Paradoxical movement is best described as chest wall movement that is
    (A) inward with both inspiration and expiration.
    (B) inward with expiration and outward with inspiration.
    (C) inward with inspiration and outward with expiration.
    (D) outward with both inspiration and expiration.

53. Prehospital management for this patient includes
    (A) a needle decompression midclavicular line.
    (B) positive pressure ventilation.
    (C) an occlusive dressing.
    (D) chest decompression midaxillary line.

54. Your patient is in severe respiratory distress. Reassessment reveals absent lung sounds on the left, tracheal deviation to the right, and a SpO_2 reading of 82%. Immediate treatment must include
    (A) intubation.
    (B) right side chest decompression.
    (C) left side chest decompression.
    (D) oxygen administration.

Questions 55–57 are based on the following scenario:

Your patient rolled a farm tractor over a hill. He has a large puncture wound to his right neck, above the clavicle. It appears that the wound is from a tree branch. Moderate bleeding is present.

55. Care for the puncture wound would include
    (A) application of direct pressure with a bulky trauma dressing.
    (B) application of an occlusive dressing.
    (C) application of a sterile dressing.
    (D) needle decompression.

56. Which transport position would be appropriate for this patient?
    (A) Trendelenburg position
    (B) Left lateral recumbent
    (C) Right lateral recumbent
    (D) Prone

57. A major concern with this type of injury is
    (A) rib fracture.
    (B) clavicle fracture.
    (C) flail chest.
    (D) edema.

---

58. Your patient is a 44-year-old female who was burned when a high-temperature water pipe exploded. She has blisters to the chest, abdomen, entire right arm, and front of the right leg. According to the rule of nines, this patient has sustained _____ percent burns.

    (A) 40.5%
    (B) 36%
    (C) 45%
    (D) 31.5%

59. You are called to a rooftop for a 17-year-old female who was sunbathing. She is alert and oriented and states she was using lotion without any SPF protection to "speed up her tan." She was in the sun from 9:00 A.M. to 2:00 P.M. She is in significant pain and requests that you help her off the rooftop. She has blisters covering the entire front of her body. You should consider this patient to have
    (A) first-degree burns.
    (B) minor burns.
    (C) nothing to worry about.
    (D) critical burns.

Questions 60 and 61 are based on the following scenario:

You respond to a "man down" call. When you arrive, you find a 52-year-old male lying on the ground next to a ladder. It is unclear if he was placing the ladder against the house when it came into contact with power lines or if he fell from the top of the ladder.

60. Examination shows the patient to be unresponsive. He has a rapid irregular pulse and snoring respirations of 8, BP is 88/42. Treatment should include
    (A) assisted ventilation with a bag-valve device at 6–10 L/min.
    (B) assisted ventilation with a nonrebreather mask at 10–15 L/min.
    (C) opening the airway with a jaw thrust maneuver and ventilation with a bag-valve device.
    (D) insertion of an oropharyngeal airway and oxygen by nonrebreather mask at 10–15 L/min.

61. You apply a cardiac monitor and note the following rhythm.

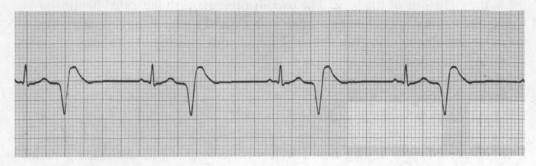

Treatment includes
(A) immediate cardioversion.
(B) immediate defibrillation.
(C) lidocaine 1 mg/kg.
(D) continued observation.

62. Which of the following facial injuries involves a fracture of both the maxillary and nasal bone?
(A) Mandibular fracture
(B) LeFort I
(C) LeFort II
(D) LeFort III

63. Cushing's reflex includes a sudden increase in systolic pressure, bradycardia, and
(A) erratic respirations.
(B) irregular pulse.
(C) increased respirations.
(D) pupil dilation.

64. Which head injury will likely result in *immediate* neurological signs/symptoms with rapid deterioration?
(A) Concussion
(B) Contusion
(C) Subdural hematoma
(D) Epidural hematoma

65. You arrive on the scene of a patient who has been stabbed with a knife in the right side of the back. The patient presents with left-sided hemiparalysis and sensory loss. Despite another stab wound to the right abdomen, the patient denies pain. What type of spinal cord injuries do you suspect?
    (A) Compression
    (B) Transection
    (C) Neurogenic shock
    (D) Brown-Sequard's syndrome

66. Which of the following best describes the effects of pericardial tamponade?
    (A) Cardiac output increases, and central venous pressure falls.
    (B) Cardiac output is reduced, and central venous pressure rises.
    (C) Cardiac output increases, and venous pressure is not affected.
    (D) Cardiac output is not affected, and central venous pressure falls.

67. Beck's triad is often associated with pericardial tamponade. It includes distant heart tones, JVD (jugular venous distension), and
    (A) pulse paradoxus.
    (B) hypotension.
    (C) wheezing.
    (D) delayed capillary refill.

68. A stab wound to the stomach or small intestine would cause gastric contents to enter the peritoneal cavity. Presentation would include
    (A) a rapid onset of cramping pain.
    (B) referred pain to the left shoulder.
    (C) a gradual onset of pain throughout the abdomen.
    (D) a rapid onset of sharp pain, diffuse throughout the abdomen.

69. Your patient was struck in the head with a six-inch-diameter tree branch while trimming a tree. He complained of dizziness immediately after the incident but states he "feels fine" now. The next day, he complains of dizziness and vomiting. You suspect a
    (A) epidural hematoma.
    (B) subdural hematoma.
    (C) concussion.
    (D) contusion.

Questions 70–73 are based on the following scenario:
You respond to an explosion at a local fireworks production factory. The explosion rocked the ground several blocks away. There are multiple patients.

70. The mechanism of injury from a blast or explosion can be from three factors; primary, secondary, and tertiary. The mechanism of injury of a patient who suffers injuries from being struck by material propelled by the blast force is considered
(A) a primary mechanism of injury.
(B) a secondary mechanism of injury.
(C) a tertiary mechanism of injury.
(D) all of the above.

71. The mechanism of injury of a patient being thrown and impacting the ground or other object is considered
(A) a primary mechanism of injury.
(B) a secondary mechanism of injury.
(C) a tertiary mechanism of injury.
(D) all of the above.

72. Your first patient is a 43-year-old male with burns over the front of his right arm, upper chest, and the front of his right leg. Using the rule of nines, what percent of burns does this patient have?
(A) 27%
(B) 22.5%
(C) 18%
(D) 35%

73. This patient is hoarse, has singed nasal hair, is coughing up charcoal-colored sputum, and has developed inspiratory stridor. Treatment should include
(A) high-flow oxygen via a simple mask.
(B) immediate endotracheal intubation.
(C) continued monitoring for complications.
(D) humidified oxygen via nasal cannula.

---

74. Which of the following statements is correct regarding a Glasgow Coma Scale score of 7?
(A) A perfect GCS score is 10 and a score of 7 represents minor injuries.
(B) A perfect GCS score is 12 and a score of 7 represents moderate injuries.
(C) A perfect GCS score is 15 and a score of 7 represents moderate injuries.
(D) A perfect GCS score is 15 and a score of 7 represents serious injuries.

Questions 75 and 76 are based on the following scenario:
You arrive on scene of a 34-year-old male who was struck by a car. Bystanders tell you the patient was standing on the sidewalk when his neighbor, who was backing out of the driveway, struck him. Your patient is sitting in the yard with an obvious open tibia/fibula fracture of the right leg.

75. As you auscultate his right upper chest, you notice the patient guarding his shoulder. Closer exam reveals a fractured clavicle. Complications associated with a fractured clavicle include injury to the
    (A) carotid artery.
    (B) subclavian vein.
    (C) descending aorta.
    (D) inferior vena cava.

76. Physical exam concludes that the right clavicle fracture and open right tibia/fibula fracture are his only obvious injuries but you are concerned because his level of consciousness is deteriorating and his heart rate has increased 30 beats per minute. Although his abdomen was unremarkable upon examination, you know that an indicator of severe abdominal trauma is the presence of
    (A) absent bowel sounds.
    (B) back pain.
    (C) referred pain to the clavicle.
    (D) unexplained shock.

---

77. There are anatomical differences in pediatric patients compared to adults. When using the rule of nines for calculating burns, which of the following is a correct modification for a child?
    (A) The front of each arm for a child is 7% compared to 4½% on an adult.
    (B) The front of each leg for a child is 4½% compared to 9% on an adult.
    (C) The head of a child is 18% compared to 9% on an adult.
    (D) The entire leg of a child is 9% compared to 18% on an adult.

Questions 78–80 are based on the following scenario:
A 22-year-old male is found in an alley with multiple stab wounds to the extremities, abdomen, and chest. BP is 82/40, pulse 142 weak, respirations 10.

78. Your exam reveals distended neck veins, equal breath sounds, and a radial pulse that disappears during inspiration. You suspect
    (A) a hemothorax.
    (B) a tension pneumothorax.
    (C) a sucking chest wound.
    (D) cardiac tamponade.

79. As you log-roll the patient to place him on the long spine board, you inspect his back and discover another stab wound just below the right scapula. You observe blood bubbling out of the wound with each breath. You suspect
    (A) a massive hemothorax.
    (B) a tension pneumothorax.
    (C) an open pneumothorax.
    (D) a hematoma formation.

80. Priority care for this patient would include
    (A) IV fluids to stabilize vital signs.
    (B) closure of the chest wall with an occlusive dressing taped on three sides.
    (C) immediate chest decompression of the right chest.
    (D) rapid transport to a trauma center.

ANSWERS AND ANSWER EXPLANATIONS

1. **(D)** Level III trauma center because it will stabilize and transfer serious patients as needed as part of a trauma system. Transport decisions will be dependent on many factors, one of those being transport time.

2. **(C)** Open the airway with a modified jaw thrust and immobilize the cervical spine. Always remember the ABCs.

3. **(B)** With the information given, hypotension, absent peripheral pulses, diminished breath sounds on the right with chest trauma on the right, a hemopneumothorax is likely.

4. **(C)** This patient received an initial assessment and rapid trauma survey to identify all life threats. It is recommended that these assessment steps be performed in two to three minutes or less.

5. **(B)** Of the choices listed, the patient with a possible head injury should be transported first. **(A)**, **(C)**, and **(D)** are all isolated injuries that do not pose an immediate life threat that a head injury is capable of.

6. **(D)** 27%—chest = 9%, abdomen = 9%, anterior surface of both arms = 9%.

7. **(D)** Manage the burns by covering them with a dry bulky dressing. A dressing reduces air movement past sensitive partial thickness burns, thus reducing pain. Damaged skin loses temperature regulation capacity so it is important to keep the patient covered, even if the environment is not cold. **(B)** is incorrect because the use of ice in any form can worsen the injury as it causes vasoconstriction and reduces blood flow to the already damaged area. **(A)** and **(C)** are incorrect because debridement or cleaning of a burn with iodine are not indicated.

8. **(B)** Current fluid resuscitation recommends that two large-bore catheters be introduced. When EMS transport time is less than one hour, a bolus of 0.5 ml of normal saline (NS) for every kilogram of the patient's weight multiplied by the percentage of BSA should be initiated.

9. **(A)** Risk factors for inhalation injuries associated with burns include standing in the burn environment (hot gases rise), screaming or yelling in the hot environment (the open glottis allows toxic gases to enter the lower airway), and being trapped in a closed burn environment.

10. **(C)** Of the choices listed, provide high-flow oxygen by nonrebreather mask at 15 liters per minute once the airway has been assured is correct. **(A)** is incorrect because it states "all" inhalation injury. **(B)** is incorrect

because the patient requires high-flow oxygen. **(D)** is incorrect because the scenario does not give you enogough information to conclude cyanide toxicity.

11. **(B)** By the time the victim of a lightning strike is reached, the electricity will have dissipated. While you may be concerned as long as the storm remains nearby, there is no danger of electrical shock from touching the victim of a lightning strike.

12. **(C)** Both acids and alkalis cause burns by disrupting cell membranes and damaging tissues on contact. **(A)** is incorrect because antidotes and neutralizing agents should never be used as they may cause a violent reaction with the contaminant. **(B)** is incorrect because alkali burns are typically more severe because of their liquefaction necrosis process. **(C)** is incorrect because you should approach from up wind.

13. **(D)** This patient is alert and oriented, so he has an intact airway and is breathing. Your priority for this patient is "circulation," which includes stopping major hemorrhage. Applying a pressure dressing and elevation are necessary. **(A)** is incorrect because it is not a higher priority than controlling hemorrhage. **(B)** is not indicated for this patient. **(C)** is incorrect because it states right leg.

14. **(B)** How well do you know your medical terminology and definitions? If you know your medical terminology you answered this question correctly because positive end expiratory pressure is not a component of essential perfusion.

15. **(A)** Once external hemorrhage has been controlled, start fluid resuscitation with normal saline (NS) or Ringer's lactate solution.

16. **(D)** Your safety is the first priority. Do not approach the car until you are notified by the proper officials that the power has been turned off.

17. **(C)** Cushing's or herniation syndrome is manifested by hypertension, bradycardia, and erratic respirations. This patient has a GCS score of 9, hypertension (178/100), bradycardia (56), and irregular respirations that indicate head injury with Cushing's syndrome.

18. **(D)** Intubation and supplemental oxygen are essential. You would hyperventilate this patient because he exhibits signs/symptoms of increased intracranial pressure (Cushing's syndrome).

19. **(A)** The objective of prehospital fluid resuscitation is to stabilize vital signs until the patient arrives at the hospital.

20. **(D)** Mechanism of injury can provide clues for determining possible injuries.

21. **(C)** Ballistics is the study of projectiles in motion. Studies suggest that wounds from rifle bullets are two to four times more lethal than handgun bullets due to mass energy and velocity.

22. **(A)** Neurogenic or distributive shock is recognized by hypotension, bradycardia, and a normal initial appearance. **(C)** is something to consider but should not be part of your initial impression. **(B)** is clearly wrong. **(D)** is incorrect because this is distributive shock not mechanical shock.

23. **(B)** You would suspect injury at the thoracic level between T4 and T11. Memorization of all of the dermatomes is difficult and really not necessary. However, you should have a general knowledge of associated injuries to the spinal nerve plexuses.

24. **(B)** The objective of prehospital fluid resuscitation is to stabilize vital signs until the patient arrives at the hospital. This patient requires close observation since neurogenic shock does not allow the body's normal compensatory mechanisms to work.

25. **(C)** Hyphema is a collection of blood in the anterior chamber of the eye due to trauma. This type of injury is a potential threat to the patient's vision and requires evaluation by an ophthalmologist.

26. **(D)** A c-spine injury should be suspected with any injury to the head. Treatment for this patient would include full body immobilization. The preferred position of transport of a hyphema is with the head elevated; therefore, you should elevate the head of the backboard.

27. **(D)** With a history of chest trauma, diminished breath sounds, agitation, increased respiratory rate, along with dusky color, you should suspect pneumothorax.

28. **(C)** The above symptoms are classic for tension pneumothorax, which is a serious and immediate life threat that requires immediate chest decompression.

29. **(C)** Priority for this patient who presents with respiratory compromise and hypovolemia is airway support and fluid resuscitation.

30. **(D)** Intestines should never be pushed back into the abdominal compartment. A moist nonadherent dressing should be gently placed over the bowel to prevent it from "drying out" because of the risk of irreversible damage.

31. **(B)** Airway and c-spine are always a priority before other treatments.

32. **(D)** As part of the normal physiologic changes with aging, a decrease occurs in brain weight and size. By the age of 80, the brain loses approximately 3.5 ounces in weight.

33. **(C)** Fluid resuscitation needs to be carefully administered due to the decreased response of the cardiovascular system with age. Reduced circulation, loss of circulatory defense responses, coupled with increased presence of ventricular dysfunction produces a significant challenge in managing shock in the elderly.

34. **(D)** Normal physiological changes to vital signs during the second trimester of pregnancy include a drop in blood pressure 10–15 mmHg due to a reduction in peripheral vascular resistance. The heart rate will increase 10–20 beats per minute due to an increased maternal blood volume. Note: The blood pressure will rise back to baseline in the third trimester. Keep these normal changes in mind when assessing a pregnant trauma patient.

35. **(A)** The backboard must be tilted on its left side 10–15 degrees to prevent supine hypotension syndrome. Tilting the board will allow the uterus to displace to the left and prevent compression of the inferior vena cava.

36. **(C)** After the third month of gestation the fetus and uterus grow rapidly. After the fifth month of pregnancy, the uterus rises out of the pelvis and is more prone to injury.

37. **(D)** Injured children can rapidly transition from a state of rapid and labored breathing to a state of total exhaustion resulting in respiratory arrest. Airway management is essential.

38. **(B)** A history of loss of consciousness is one of the most important prognostic indicators of potential CNS injury.

39. **(A)** Contrary to popular belief, pulse oximetry is not the "fifth vital sign." Complete documentation of baseline neurological status includes response to sensory stimulation, pupillary reaction, and motor function.

40. **(B)** Positive pressure ventilation of the patient with a flail chest injury reverses the mechanism that causes the paradoxical chest wall movement, restores tidal volume, and reduces pain of chest wall movement.

41. **(B)** The amount of energy required to deform a steering wheel is significant. Possible life-threatening injuries from the body striking a steering wheel include: flail chest, myocardial contusion, aortic tear, tracheal or vascular injuries, pulmonary contusion, pneumothorax, solid and hollow

organ injury. Bilateral femur fractures may result if an "up-and-over" path occurred.

42. **(D)** Alcohol is a central nervous system depressant. Because of this, alcohol can mask signs and symptoms of injury. It is important to assess all trauma patients thoroughly, but be especially meticulous when you suspect drug/alcohol use.

43. **(B)** Osteoporosis is common in the geriatric population. This disease process makes bones much more susceptible to hip and other fractures. In severe cases, a simple action such as sneezing may result in a fracture.

44. **(C)** Crushing syndrome is a complex process. Part of this process causes toxin production including an increased potassium level. One of the major concerns with releasing a body part that has been crushed for several hours is the release of toxins into the circulating blood volume, which can lead to cardiac arrhythmia and immediate death.

45. **(D)** Crushing syndrome creates lactic acid due to anaerobic metabolism that takes place within the crushed body part. One of the major concerns with releasing a body part that has been crushed for several hours is the release of the lactic acid and other toxins into the circulating blood volume that can lead to profound metabolic acidosis. Sodium bicarbonate is indicated in the treatment of Crushing syndrome.

46. **(A)** Rupture of the stomach or small bowel that allows digestive enzymes to enter the peritoneal cavity can cause peritonitis, which can lead to infection and serious complications.

47. **(B)** Stabilizing the machinery serves two purposes. First, it assures your safety, and second it will prevent additional injury to the patient. If you choose "control bleeding" for your answer (C), this is important but it does not supersede *your* safety. (C) and (D) will both be done, but *after* the machinery is stabilized.

48. **(B)** This patient is in compensated shock. His elevated pulse rate (142) and evidence of vasoconstriction (pale, moist skin) is able to maintain his blood pressure despite continued blood loss.

49. **(B)** If bleeding still persists after direct pressure and elevation, the next step is to find an arterial pulse point proximal to the wound and apply firm pressure.

50. **(A)** Decompensated shock is when the body can no longer respond to the continued blood loss. This is evident in the scenario by a decreased pulse rate, respirations, and blood pressure.

51. **(C)** Flail chest is three or more adjacent ribs that are fractured in two or more places. This segment of the chest is free to move with the pressure changes of respirations.

52. **(C)** Paradoxical chest wall movement associated with flail chest is defined as the motion of a flail segment opposite to the normal motion of the chest wall.

53. **(B)** Positive pressure ventilation of the patient with a flail chest reverses the mechanism that causes the paradoxical chest wall movement, restores tidal volume, and reduces the pain of chest wall movement.

54. **(C)** The signs and symptoms displayed by this patient are consistent with a left side tension pneumothorax and immediate chest decompression is required.

55. **(B)** Application of an occlusive dressing is necessary because this is a highly vascular area. An occlusive dressing will prevent air from entering an injured vessel and the development of an air embolism.

56. **(A)** The Trendelenburg position would be appropriate to decrease the potential for air aspiration into an injured vessel.

57. **(D)** Edema is a serious concern because injury to this highly vascular area of the neck can lead to a rapidly expanding hematoma. This hematoma can put pressure on other blood vessels resulting in decreased blood flow to the brain or put pressure on nearby airway structures resulting in an airway management nightmare!

58. **(B)** 36%—chest = 9%, abdomen = 9%, entire arm 9%, front of the leg = 9%.

59. **(D)** This should be classified as a critical burn with over 50% body surface area containing second-degree burns.

60. **(C)** It is unclear if this patient fell, so you must suspect trauma and c-spine injury. A jaw thrust maneuver and bag-valve mask ventilation is the best choice. **(A)** is incorrect because the oxygen flow setting is too low; it should be at least 15 L/min. **(B)** is incorrect because it utilizes a nonrebreather mask to assist ventilations. Nonrebreathers are not designed for or capable of assisting ventilations. **(D)** is incorrect because the patient needs his ventilations assisted.

61. **(C)** Treatment for this rhythm includes lidocaine 1 mg/kg IVP.

62. (C) This is a difficult question. If you knew this answer, pat yourself on the back. A LeFort II fracture involves both the maxillary and nasal bones.

63. (A) Cushing's reflex includes an increase in systolic blood pressure, bradycardia, and erratic (usually slow) respirations.

64. (D) An epidural hematoma involves arterial vessels. Because the bleeding is arterial, intracranial pressure builds rapidly, compressing the cerebrum and increasing pressure within the skull. As the pressure rapidly builds, the patient will immediately display neurological signs/symptoms.

65. (D) This is another difficult question. If you knew this answer, pat yourself on the back. Brown-Sequard's syndrome is caused by a penetrating injury that affects one side of the spinal cord. The damage to the one side results in sensory and motor loss to that side of the body. Pain and temperature perception are lost on the opposite side of the body because of the switching of the associated nerves as they enter the spinal cord.

66. (B) In pericardial tamponade, the pericardial sac fills with fluid and compresses the heart. This impairs ventricular filling. The result is a decrease in cardiac output (the left ventricle cannot effectively fill and pump) and an increase in central venous pressure (venous blood returning to the heart is impaired and the right ventricle cannot fill or pump effectively).

67. (B) Beck's triad includes hypotension, distant heart tones, and JVD. This triad of symptoms can aid in the diagnosis of cardiac tamponade.

68. (D) Injury to the stomach or small bowel that allows digestive enzymes to enter the peritoneal cavity can cause a rapid development of sharp pain throughout the abdomen. This is a serious concern because peritonitis can develop and lead to serious complications.

69. (B) A subdural hematoma is usually due to rupture of small venous vessels. This type of bleeding is slow and the onset of symptoms may take several hours to develop after the injury.

70. (B) A secondary mechanism of injury from a blast or explosion is defined as any injury sustained from being struck by material propelled by the blast force.

71. (C) A tertiary mechanism of injury from a blast or explosion is defined as any injury sustained from being thrown and impacting the ground or other objects.

72. (B) 22.5%—front of right arm = 4.5%, upper chest = 9%, front of right leg = 9%.

73. **(B)** Your concern with this patient is complete airway obstruction secondary to swelling of the airway. Immediate endotracheal intubation is indicated.

74. **(D)** A perfect GCS score is 15. A score between 9 and 12 indicates moderate injury, while a score of 8 or below represents severe head injury.

75. **(B)** Complications associated with a fracture of the clavicle include injury to the subclavian vein.

76. **(D)** When assessment of a trauma patient does not reveal significant injury, the presence of unexplained shock should lead you to suspect serious abdominal/thorax trauma.

77. **(C)** When using the rule of nines, the head of a child is assigned 18% BSA compared to 9% BSA on an adult. There are several other "rule of nine" modifications for children and infants you should be familiar with before taking your certification exam.

78. **(D)** The diagnosis of cardiac tamponade often relies upon symptoms. Hypotension, distended neck veins, and muffled heart sounds are classic symptoms of cardiac tamponade and are known as Beck's triad. If the patient loses his or her peripheral pulse during inspiration, it is suggestive of pulsus paradoxus and the presence of cardiac tamponade.

79. **(C)** An open pneumothorax (sucking chest wound) includes a sucking or bubbling sound as air moves in and out of the chest wall. Bleeding is usually present and frothing of the blood may occur as the air and blood combine.

80. **(B)** Treatment of an open pneumothorax includes closing the chest wall by application of an occlusive dressing that is taped on three sides. **(A)** may be necessary, but it is not a more important priority than sealing the chest. **(D)** is necessary for this patient but sealing the chest should be performed on-scene, prior to rapid transport to a trauma center. **(C)** is incorrect because this patient does not have a tension pneumothorax although he will need to be monitored closely because an open pneumothorax can rapidly transition into a tension pneumothorax.

Notes

Obstetrics/Gynecology/ Pediatrics

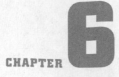

This chapter has 45 questions devoted to obstetrics and gynecology, with the remaining 75 questions devoted to pediatric emergencies.

It is essential that you know pediatric drug dosages. If you are guessing the answers for these questions, STOP!! While you have the luxury of thinking about (and guessing) the answer to these questions as you go through this chapter, you will not have that luxury when you have a patient in front of you. You *must* know the correct dosage!

All ECG rhythm strips used in this chapter are six-second strips.

Answer Sheet
CHAPTER 6—OBSTETRICS/ GYNECOLOGY/PEDIATRICS

1 Ⓐ Ⓑ Ⓒ Ⓓ	31 Ⓐ Ⓑ Ⓒ Ⓓ	61 Ⓐ Ⓑ Ⓒ Ⓓ	91 Ⓐ Ⓑ Ⓒ Ⓓ
2 Ⓐ Ⓑ Ⓒ Ⓓ	32 Ⓐ Ⓑ Ⓒ Ⓓ	62 Ⓐ Ⓑ Ⓒ Ⓓ	92 Ⓐ Ⓑ Ⓒ Ⓓ
3 Ⓐ Ⓑ Ⓒ Ⓓ	33 Ⓐ Ⓑ Ⓒ Ⓓ	63 Ⓐ Ⓑ Ⓒ Ⓓ	93 Ⓐ Ⓑ Ⓒ Ⓓ
4 Ⓐ Ⓑ Ⓒ Ⓓ	34 Ⓐ Ⓑ Ⓒ Ⓓ	64 Ⓐ Ⓑ Ⓒ Ⓓ	94 Ⓐ Ⓑ Ⓒ Ⓓ
5 Ⓐ Ⓑ Ⓒ Ⓓ	35 Ⓐ Ⓑ Ⓒ Ⓓ	65 Ⓐ Ⓑ Ⓒ Ⓓ	95 Ⓐ Ⓑ Ⓒ Ⓓ
6 Ⓐ Ⓑ Ⓒ Ⓓ	36 Ⓐ Ⓑ Ⓒ Ⓓ	66 Ⓐ Ⓑ Ⓒ Ⓓ	96 Ⓐ Ⓑ Ⓒ Ⓓ
7 Ⓐ Ⓑ Ⓒ Ⓓ	37 Ⓐ Ⓑ Ⓒ Ⓓ	67 Ⓐ Ⓑ Ⓒ Ⓓ	97 Ⓐ Ⓑ Ⓒ Ⓓ
8 Ⓐ Ⓑ Ⓒ Ⓓ	38 Ⓐ Ⓑ Ⓒ Ⓓ	68 Ⓐ Ⓑ Ⓒ Ⓓ	98 Ⓐ Ⓑ Ⓒ Ⓓ
9 Ⓐ Ⓑ Ⓒ Ⓓ	39 Ⓐ Ⓑ Ⓒ Ⓓ	69 Ⓐ Ⓑ Ⓒ Ⓓ	99 Ⓐ Ⓑ Ⓒ Ⓓ
10 Ⓐ Ⓑ Ⓒ Ⓓ	40 Ⓐ Ⓑ Ⓒ Ⓓ	70 Ⓐ Ⓑ Ⓒ Ⓓ	100 Ⓐ Ⓑ Ⓒ Ⓓ
11 Ⓐ Ⓑ Ⓒ Ⓓ	41 Ⓐ Ⓑ Ⓒ Ⓓ	71 Ⓐ Ⓑ Ⓒ Ⓓ	101 Ⓐ Ⓑ Ⓒ Ⓓ
12 Ⓐ Ⓑ Ⓒ Ⓓ	42 Ⓐ Ⓑ Ⓒ Ⓓ	72 Ⓐ Ⓑ Ⓒ Ⓓ	102 Ⓐ Ⓑ Ⓒ Ⓓ
13 Ⓐ Ⓑ Ⓒ Ⓓ	43 Ⓐ Ⓑ Ⓒ Ⓓ	73 Ⓐ Ⓑ Ⓒ Ⓓ	103 Ⓐ Ⓑ Ⓒ Ⓓ
14 Ⓐ Ⓑ Ⓒ Ⓓ	44 Ⓐ Ⓑ Ⓒ Ⓓ	74 Ⓐ Ⓑ Ⓒ Ⓓ	104 Ⓐ Ⓑ Ⓒ Ⓓ
15 Ⓐ Ⓑ Ⓒ Ⓓ	45 Ⓐ Ⓑ Ⓒ Ⓓ	75 Ⓐ Ⓑ Ⓒ Ⓓ	105 Ⓐ Ⓑ Ⓒ Ⓓ
16 Ⓐ Ⓑ Ⓒ Ⓓ	46 Ⓐ Ⓑ Ⓒ Ⓓ	76 Ⓐ Ⓑ Ⓒ Ⓓ	106 Ⓐ Ⓑ Ⓒ Ⓓ
17 Ⓐ Ⓑ Ⓒ Ⓓ	47 Ⓐ Ⓑ Ⓒ Ⓓ	77 Ⓐ Ⓑ Ⓒ Ⓓ	107 Ⓐ Ⓑ Ⓒ Ⓓ
18 Ⓐ Ⓑ Ⓒ Ⓓ	48 Ⓐ Ⓑ Ⓒ Ⓓ	78 Ⓐ Ⓑ Ⓒ Ⓓ	108 Ⓐ Ⓑ Ⓒ Ⓓ
19 Ⓐ Ⓑ Ⓒ Ⓓ	49 Ⓐ Ⓑ Ⓒ Ⓓ	79 Ⓐ Ⓑ Ⓒ Ⓓ	109 Ⓐ Ⓑ Ⓒ Ⓓ
20 Ⓐ Ⓑ Ⓒ Ⓓ	50 Ⓐ Ⓑ Ⓒ Ⓓ	80 Ⓐ Ⓑ Ⓒ Ⓓ	110 Ⓐ Ⓑ Ⓒ Ⓓ
21 Ⓐ Ⓑ Ⓒ Ⓓ	51 Ⓐ Ⓑ Ⓒ Ⓓ	81 Ⓐ Ⓑ Ⓒ Ⓓ	111 Ⓐ Ⓑ Ⓒ Ⓓ
22 Ⓐ Ⓑ Ⓒ Ⓓ	52 Ⓐ Ⓑ Ⓒ Ⓓ	82 Ⓐ Ⓑ Ⓒ Ⓓ	112 Ⓐ Ⓑ Ⓒ Ⓓ
23 Ⓐ Ⓑ Ⓒ Ⓓ	53 Ⓐ Ⓑ Ⓒ Ⓓ	83 Ⓐ Ⓑ Ⓒ Ⓓ	113 Ⓐ Ⓑ Ⓒ Ⓓ
24 Ⓐ Ⓑ Ⓒ Ⓓ	54 Ⓐ Ⓑ Ⓒ Ⓓ	84 Ⓐ Ⓑ Ⓒ Ⓓ	114 Ⓐ Ⓑ Ⓒ Ⓓ
25 Ⓐ Ⓑ Ⓒ Ⓓ	55 Ⓐ Ⓑ Ⓒ Ⓓ	85 Ⓐ Ⓑ Ⓒ Ⓓ	115 Ⓐ Ⓑ Ⓒ Ⓓ
26 Ⓐ Ⓑ Ⓒ Ⓓ	56 Ⓐ Ⓑ Ⓒ Ⓓ	86 Ⓐ Ⓑ Ⓒ Ⓓ	116 Ⓐ Ⓑ Ⓒ Ⓓ
27 Ⓐ Ⓑ Ⓒ Ⓓ	57 Ⓐ Ⓑ Ⓒ Ⓓ	87 Ⓐ Ⓑ Ⓒ Ⓓ	117 Ⓐ Ⓑ Ⓒ Ⓓ
28 Ⓐ Ⓑ Ⓒ Ⓓ	58 Ⓐ Ⓑ Ⓒ Ⓓ	88 Ⓐ Ⓑ Ⓒ Ⓓ	118 Ⓐ Ⓑ Ⓒ Ⓓ
29 Ⓐ Ⓑ Ⓒ Ⓓ	59 Ⓐ Ⓑ Ⓒ Ⓓ	89 Ⓐ Ⓑ Ⓒ Ⓓ	119 Ⓐ Ⓑ Ⓒ Ⓓ
30 Ⓐ Ⓑ Ⓒ Ⓓ	60 Ⓐ Ⓑ Ⓒ Ⓓ	90 Ⓐ Ⓑ Ⓒ Ⓓ	120 Ⓐ Ⓑ Ⓒ Ⓓ

1. Supine hypotension syndrome occurs from
   (A) reduction of cardiac output due to compression of the aorta.
   (B) reduction of cardiac output due to compression of the inferior vena cava.
   (C) reduction of cardiac output due to compression of the superior vena cava.
   (D) the uterus pushing up on the diaphragm.

2. You are caring for a female patient who is at 35 weeks gestation. She was involved in a car accident and complains of neck pain. You suspect spinal injury and fully immobilize her on a long spine board. You would then
   (A) carefully tilt the board on its left side 10–15 degrees.
   (B) carefully tilt the board on its right side 10–15 degrees.
   (C) manually displace the uterus to the right.
   (D) allow the patient to roll onto her side.

3. The major concern with a prolapsed cord is that it
   (A) will dry, become contaminated, and infection may result.
   (B) will delay delivery.
   (C) will be compressed and reduce blood flow to the infant, resulting in hypoxia.
   (D) will lower the temperature of the blood going to the infant, when exposed to room temperature.

4. Abdominal pain in the region of the ovary during ovulation is known as
   (A) Braxton-Hicks contractions.
   (B) cystitis.
   (C) mittelschmerz.
   (D) endometritis.

5. In obstetrics, a woman's parity refers to her number of
   (A) pregnancies.
   (B) viable deliveries.
   (C) cesarean sections.
   (D) spontaneous abortions.

6. Your patient is 26 years old and 30 weeks pregnant. She complains of sudden severe tearing abdominal pain with some minor vaginal bleeding. Upon careful palpation, her abdomen is very tender and her uterus seems to be tightly contracted. You suspect
   (A) abruptio placenta.
   (B) an ectopic pregnancy.
   (C) a miscarriage.
   (D) placenta previa.

7. Placenta abruption is a medical emergency caused by
   (A) implantation of the fertilized ovum in a fallopian tube.
   (B) the uterus covering the cervical opening.
   (C) premature separation of the placenta from the uterine wall.
   (D) spontaneous abortion.

8. A multigravida and nullipara pregnancy history includes
   (A) one pregnancy and one birth.
   (B) many pregnancies and one birth.
   (C) one pregnancy and no births.
   (D) many pregnancies and no births.

9. Which of the following best states the normal physiological changes to vital signs during the second trimester of pregnancy?
   (A) Blood pressure rises, pulse rate rises
   (B) Blood pressure rises, pulse rate falls
   (C) Blood pressure falls, pulse rate rises
   (D) Blood pressure falls, pulse rate falls

10. Signs and symptoms of a pregnant patient with preeclampsia include
    (A) elevated BP, increased weight gain, facial edema, and seizures.
    (B) elevated BP, abdominal rigidity, and bright red vaginal bleeding.
    (C) elevated BP, normal respirations, and normal pulse rate.
    (D) elevated BP, visual disturbance, headache, and edema.

Questions 11–14 are based on the following scenario:

You are called to the scene of a 26-year-old female patient who is 27 weeks pregnant and in active labor. The patient states, "The baby is coming." You perform a visual examination of the perineum and notice a prolapsed cord.

11. You would immediately place the patient in which position?
    (A) Hips elevated as much as possible
    (B) Knee-chest position
    (C) Left lateral recumbent position
    (D) Both A and B are correct

12. You would instruct the patient to
    (A) push with each contraction.
    (B) pant with each contraction.
    (C) bear down.
    (D) hold her breath.

13. Additional treatment would include
    (A) providing oxygen and preparing to assist the mother for a normal delivery.
    (B) with a gloved hand, attempting to push the cord back into the vagina, and transporting with lights and siren.
    (C) with a gloved hand, placing two fingers into the vagina to raise the fetus off the cord, providing oxygen and transport.
    (D) attempting to reposition the cord laterally by gently pulling on it.

14. Care for the prolapsed cord would include
    (A) application of a sterile dressing.
    (B) attempting to reposition the cord.
    (C) doing nothing.
    (D) packing in ice to prevent it from drying.

---

15. The hormone secreted by the pituitary gland that stimulates the uterus to produce stronger contractions is
    (A) estrogen.
    (B) actin.
    (C) progesterone.
    (D) oxytocin.

16. The most common sexually transmitted disease is
    (A) chlamydia.
    (B) gonorrhea.
    (C) syphilis.
    (D) herpes.

17. You are treating a 20-year-old female complaining of abdominal pain that becomes more intense when walking. She states that if she shuffles her feet when she walks, the pain isn't as intense. Other signs and symptoms include fever, chills, and nausea. This patient is most likely suffering from
    (A) endometritis.
    (B) pelvic inflammatory disease.
    (C) ruptured ovarian cyst.
    (D) mittelschmerz cystitis.

Questions 18–20 are based on the following scenario:

You are called to a 32-year-old female who is in her twenty-eighth week of pregnancy. She complains of dizziness, blurred vision, and a feeling that she is going to pass out. She is emotionally upset and crying. At her doctor's appointment last week, her doctor scolded her for gaining too much weight. Her hands and ankles are edematous and her face is puffy. Vitals are BP 178/108, pulse 104, respirations 24.

18. You suspect that this patient
    (A) is emotionally upset.
    (B) has preeclampsia.
    (C) has borderline hypotension.
    (D) has postpartum depression.

19. Treatment for this patient would include
    (A) rapid transport with lights and siren.
    (B) administering nitroglycerin to lower the blood pressure.
    (C) transporting for psychiatric evaluation.
    (D) keeping the patient calm, and transporting without lights and siren.

20. You are enroute to the hospital when the patient has a grand mal seizure. Treatment for this patient includes
    (A) administering high-flow oxygen, magnesium sulfate 2–5 mg.
    (B) administering oxygen, magnesium sulfate 2–5 g, placing her in right lateral recumbent position.
    (C) maintaining an airway, administering oxygen, administering magnesium sulfate 2–5 g, monitoring vital signs.
    (D) maintaining an airway, administering magnesium sulfate 6–8 g, monitoring vital signs, placing her in left lateral recumbent position.

Questions 21 and 22 are based on the following scenario:

Your patient is a 38-year-old multigravida in her thirtieth week of gestation. She presents with bright red vaginal bleeding but denies abdominal pain. Her uterus is soft and feels "out of place." Her problem began following sexual intercourse.

21. You suspect
    (A) a uterine rupture.
    (B) placenta previa.
    (C) an ectopic pregnancy.
    (D) abruptio placenta.

22. Management of this patient includes all of the following except
    (A) IV fluids.
    (B) high-flow oxygen.
    (C) a vaginal examination.
    (D) transport for evaluation.

---

23. APGAR assessment of a newborn should be performed

    (A) only in the ambulance during transport.
    (B) at one and five minutes after birth.
    (C) at five-minute intervals after birth.
    (D) immediately after delivery and then every two minutes.

24. If the amniotic sac has not ruptured and the baby's head emerges, you should
    (A) use a sterile scalpel to carefully open the sac and provide suction before the baby takes a breath.
    (B) delay further delivery and transport immediately for an emergency cesarean section.
    (C) use your fingers to pinch and puncture the sac, then push the sac away from the nose and mouth.
    (D) continue with the delivery; the sac will break on its own once the baby's head is delivered.

25. Suctioning of the infant's mouth and nose should be performed after
    (A) the cord is clamped and cut.
    (B) the infant begins to cry.
    (C) the chest has been delivered.
    (D) the head has been delivered.

26. Chest compressions should be performed on any newborn with a heart rate less than ___ beats per minute.
    (A) 60
    (B) 40
    (C) 100
    (D) 120

27. Your 26-year-old female patient complains of nausea, dizziness, sudden onset of sharp left lower quadrant pain, and shoulder pain. You suspect
    (A) a ruptured appendix.
    (B) an ectopic pregnancy.
    (C) cholecystitis.
    (D) kidney stones.

28. The function of the placenta includes all of the following except
    (A) the transfer of antibodies.
    (B) the transfer of oxygen and nutrients.
    (C) the production of hormones.
    (D) the excretion of CO_2 and waste products.

29. Which of the following is the most appropriate care for a suspected sexual assault patient?
    (A) Perform a limited physical examination and care for injuries requiring immediate treatment.
    (B) Conduct a SAMPLE history and have the patient bathe prior to transporting to the hospital.
    (C) Prior to transport examine the genitalia for signs of injury.
    (D) Have the patient remove all clothing and place all clothing in a plastic bag.

Questions 30 and 31 are based on the following scenario:

You arrive on the scene of a 25-year-old female who states she is 9 months pregnant and is in apparent labor. The patient states she is gravida 3, para 2. She states that her "water broke" about 15 minutes ago and the baby is coming. Vital signs are: BP 152/86, pulse 96, respirations 24.

30. The term "gravida" means
    (A) number of live children.
    (B) number of pregnancies.
    (C) number of miscarriages.
    (D) time period for intrauterine fetal development.

31. Upon visual examination, you notice that crowning is present. You should
    (A) place the patient in the right lateral recumbent position and transport.
    (B) prepare for delivery because the birth of the baby is imminent.
    (C) place the patient in the knee to chest position and transport with lights and siren.
    (D) place the patient on her left side; birth of the baby will be delayed.

Questions 32 and 33 are based on the following scenario:
You arrive on the scene of a motor vehicle crash and notice that a car has struck a telephone pole. There is extensive damage to the vehicle. You find a confused female in her mid-twenties complaining of neck, chest, and abdominal pain. She keeps asking if her baby is going to be okay. You find out that she is eight months pregnant. Assessment reveals a large laceration to the forehead with active bleeding, BP 96/54, pulse 142, with pale cool skin, respirations 24 and shallow.

32. Treatment includes
    (A) placing the patient on 100% oxygen, continuing your assessment, immobilizing to the KED, transporting.
    (B) immediately removing the patient onto a backboard, administering 100% oxygen, starting two large-bore IVs, placing her on a backboard 30 degrees on the left side, and transporting.
    (C) administering 100% oxygen, rapid extrication from the vehicle with c-spine immobilization onto a backboard, placing her on a backboard on the left side, starting two large-bore IVs while enroute to the hospital.
    (D) removing the patient from the vehicle while protecting the c-spine, immobilizing the patient on the backboard and placing her in the right lateral recumbent position, administering high-flow oxygen, gaining IV access enroute to the hospital.

33. During transport, she suddenly goes into cardiac arrest. The patient is apneic and pulseless and the cardiac monitor shows ventricular fibrillation. What should be your next action?
    (A) intubate the trachea and confirm tube placement, chest compressions, administer epinephrine 1 mg every 3 to 5 minutes, rapid transport to the hospital.
    (B) defibrillate, begin CPR and intubate, administer epinephrine 1 mg IVP.
    (C) defibrillate, begin CPR, administer amiodarone 150 mg IVP.
    (D) stop resuscitative measures since this was blunt trauma and there is no chance of survival.

34. You are treating a 22-year-old female complaining of severe abdominal pain and left shoulder pain. Vital signs are BP 88/64, pulse 128 and regular, respirations of 22, skin cool and wet. She states that she has a small amount of pink vaginal discharge. This patient is most likely experiencing
    (A) a ruptured ectopic pregnancy.
    (B) endometriosis.
    (C) pelvic inflammatory disease.
    (D) amenorrhea.

35. You are providing positive-pressure ventilation to a newborn. Which of the following statements is correct regarding oxygen administration to a newborn?
    (A) An anesthesia bag provides the best ventilation and is easiest to use.
    (B) A large bag-valve is needed to provide adequate tidal volume.
    (C) Never deprive a newborn of oxygen for fear of oxygen toxicity.
    (D) Positive pressure ventilations are often required in newborn resuscitation.

36. To prevent over- or undertransfusion of blood from the umbilical cord to the newborn, correct positioning of the newborn until the umbilical cord is clamped should be
    (A) at the level of the vagina.
    (B) at a higher level than the placenta.
    (C) at a level lower than the vagina.
    (D) placed in the left lateral recumbent position.

37. The umbilical vein
    (A) carries fetal blood to the placenta.
    (B) carries oxygenated blood from the placenta to the fetus.
    (C) returns oxygenated blood from the fetus to the placenta.
    (D) produces testosterone for male newborns and estrogen for female infants.

38. Four assessment maneuvers used to determine fetal position is called
    (A) the Leopold maneuver.
    (B) passive movement.
    (C) the Lewis manipulation.
    (D) the Patterson maneuver.

39. Contraction intervals are correctly measured
    (A) from the beginning of one contraction to the end.
    (B) from the end of one contraction to the end of the next.
    (C) from the beginning of one contraction to the beginning of the next.
    (D) from the end of one contraction to the beginning of the next.

40. Contraction length is correctly measured
    (A) from the beginning of one contraction to the end.
    (B) from the end of one contraction to the end of the next.
    (C) from the beginning of one contraction to the beginning of the next.
    (D) from the end of one contraction to the beginning of the next.

41. You have a female patient at 39 weeks' gestation. She has regular contractions lasting 45–60 seconds at one- to two-minute intervals and is crowning. Treatment for this patient should include
    (A) transport since delivery will not occur immediately.
    (B) preparing for delivery.
    (C) starting immediate transport to the hospital.
    (D) placing the patient on her left side and administering oxygen.

42. You are delivering a child when you observe the umbilical cord wrapped around the neck. Your first action should be
    (A) to stop delivery and delay as long as possible.
    (B) to gently remove the cord from around the neck.
    (C) to immediately cut the cord and remove it from around the neck.
    (D) rapid transport to the delivery room.

43. You are delivering a child in a breech presentation. You have delivered the feet and chest. You note that the chest of the child is moving and suspect the child is attempting to breathe. You should
    (A) guide the body toward the floor to assist in delivering the head.
    (B) gently pull on the torso to allow the head to be delivered.
    (C) insert two fingers in the vagina to form an airway around the infant's nose and mouth.
    (D) instruct the mother to pant with her next contraction.

44. Applying gentle countertraction to the infant's head to prevent explosive delivery is essential because
    (A) fetal hypoxia can result from rapid delivery.
    (B) if a nuchal cord is present, rapid delivery will make it worse.
    (C) this will allow the perineum to stretch and reduce the chance of tearing.
    (D) the placenta will detach too soon in rapid delivery.

45. Meconium-stained amniotic fluid indicates
    (A) a fetal hypoxic incident.
    (B) that the infant is full term.
    (C) no concern.
    (D) low birth weight.

Questions 46 and 47 are based on the following scenario:

You are sent to a private residence for a 13-month-old child with a barky cough. He is awake, slow to respond, and visibly uncomfortable. The barky cough is audible without a stethoscope but lung sounds reveal inspiratory stridor at rest. There is use of accessory muscles and you note nasal flaring.

46. You would suspect the child to be suffering from
    (A) epiglottitis.
    (B) croup.
    (C) bronchiolitis.
    (D) a common cold.

47. This child can be categorized as a child who is experiencing
    (A) respiratory arrest.
    (B) respiratory insufficiency.
    (C) prerespiratory arrest.
    (D) respiratory failure.

---

48. You are treating a 50 kg child who was found to be unconscious. The cardiac monitor attached to the patient shows a heart rate of 200 beats per minute with narrow QRS complexes. You palpate a weak pulse; blood pressure is 60/32. Oxygen is being delivered and an IV line has been established. Initial management of this patient would include

    (A) giving Adenocard 6 mg IVP.
    (B) synchronizing cardioversion at 25 joules.
    (C) synchronizing cardioversion at 100 joules.
    (D) transporting with continued assessment.

49. The recommended pediatric dose of naloxone for infants and children from birth to five years is
    (A) 20 mg.
    (B) 2.0 mg.
    (C) 0.01 mg/kg.
    (D) 0.1 mg/kg.

50. You are transporting a seven-year-old male who has sustained multisystem trauma. Appropriate administration of fluid would be to
    (A) rapidly infuse 250–300 cc of dextrose 5% in water.
    (B) rapidly infuse 350 cc of dextrose 5% in water.
    (C) determine the child's weight in kilograms and administer a 20 cc/kg bolus of an isotonic crystalloid.
    (D) give an immediate rapid infusion of normal saline, reassess, and then give additional boluses as needed.

51. You have been called to treat a five-year-old child previously diagnosed with an upper respiratory infection. She now presents with increased work of breathing, fever, and increased cough. The child appears pale, is lying on the couch, and slow to respond. She has obvious nasal flaring with a respiratory rate of eight per minute. This child is most likely in
    (A) respiratory distress with impending respiratory failure.
    (B) no acute distress.
    (C) respiratory insufficiency easily corrected with oxygen.
    (D) cardiogenic shock.

52. The MOST appropriate endotracheal tube for a 6-year-old child is
    (A) 4.0 mm, cuffed.
    (B) 4.5 mm, cuffed.
    (C) 5.0 mm, uncuffed.
    (D) 5.5 mm, uncuffed.

53. Signs and symptoms associated with shaken baby syndrome might include
    (A) contusions or abrasions visible on the knees of children three to five years old.
    (B) an intracranial hemorrhage resulting from torn veins between the brain and skull in children under the age of 24 months.
    (C) a red rash visible on the child's chest and back.
    (D) a spiral fracture of the wrist.

54. You respond to a call for a two-month-old female who is reported by the mother to be seizing. Upon arrival, you find the infant lying in a crib motionless; no seizure activity is evident. The mother reports that the episode began approximately 10 minutes ago. Your assessment reveals a flaccid infant with slow respirations of 10 per minute; bulging anterior fontanel, and several areas of bruising on the extremities in various stages of healing. From the information given and the general appearance of the infant, you suspect
    (A) child abuse, most probably shaken baby syndrome.
    (B) respiratory insufficiency with shock.
    (C) cardiovascular compromise with impending arrest.
    (D) a postictal state.

55. You are assessing a newborn infant who presents with respiratory distress. Physical findings reveal that the patient has a low birth weight, a small head, and small eye openings. Besides the obvious respiratory distress, you might suspect the infant to be suffering from
    (A) a heroin overdose.
    (B) crack cocaine ingestion.
    (C) fetal alcohol syndrome.
    (D) apnea of infancy.

56. You are assessing a 1½-year-old male who presents with obvious breathing difficulty. Inspiratory stridor is heard with evident use of all accessory muscles. The trouble breathing is worse at night. No other significant findings are visible. The child is on no medications and has otherwise been well. You suspect
    (A) epiglottitis.
    (B) asthma.
    (C) bronchiolitis.
    (D) croup.

57. Intraosseous access allows for the administration of fluids, medications, and blood products into the bone marrow. Possible complications of intraosseous infusion include all of the following except
    (A) osteomyelitis.
    (B) improvement in vascular volume and/or condition.
    (C) fractures.
    (D) compartment syndrome.

58. When caring for a pediatric patient, the standard dose of epinephrine for pulseless arrest or symptomatic bradycardia is
    (A) 0.1 mg/kg IV/IO of 1:1,000.
    (B) 0.01 mg/kg IV/IO of 1:10,000.
    (C) 0.01 mg/kg IV/IO of 1:1,000.
    (D) 0.1 mg/kg IV/IO of 1:10,000.

59. The recommended dose of amiodarone in a pediatric patient with ventricular fibrillation is
    (A) 5 mg.
    (B) 150 mg.
    (C) 0.5 mg/kg.
    (D) 5 mg/kg.

60. A ___ orogastric tube would the MOST appropriate size for a 4-year-old child.
    (A) 4F
    (B) 6F
    (C) 8F
    (D) 10F

61. When performing two-rescuer infant CPR, you should
    (A) deliver at least 120 compressions per minute.
    (B) perform a compression-to-ventilation ratio of 15:2.
    (C) reassess for a palpable brachial pulse every 5 minutes.
    (D) allow partial chest recoil in between each compression.

62. During your assessment of a five-year-old child, you discover a heart rate of 200 beats per minute. The rhythm strip reveals narrow QRS complexes corresponding to the patient's pulse rate. The rhythm most probably represents
    (A) ventricular tachycardia.
    (B) rapid atrial fibrillation.
    (C) supraventricular tachycardia.
    (D) sinus tachycardia.

63. Management of pediatric bradycardia with significant signs and symptoms related to cardiac or respiratory compromise should be treated with
    (A) atropine.
    (B) lidocaine.
    (C) sodium bicarbonate.
    (D) epinephrine.

64. Which of the following statements regarding one-rescuer child CPR is correct?
    (A) Compress the chest one half to two thirds its total depth.
    (B) Coordinate compressions and ventilations in a 15:2 ratio.
    (C) Allow the chest to recoil fully between compressions.
    (D) Reassess for pulse/breathing after 5 cycles of CPR.

65. The MOST appropriate vagal maneuver for an infant in SVT involves
    (A) blowing into an occluded straw.
    (B) holding ice packs firmly to the face.
    (C) firmly massaging the carotid artery.
    (D) encouraging the infant to bear down.

66. Hemodynamically stable children with wide QRS complex tachycardia
    (A) should receive amiodarone.
    (B) respond well to adenosine.
    (C) are likely experiencing SVT.
    (D) will respond to vagal maneuvers.

67. The recommended dose of lidocaine in the pediatric cardiac arrest patient presenting in ventricular fibrillation is
    (A) 0.001 mg/kg.
    (B) 0.01–0.02 mg/kg.
    (C) 0.1–0.2 mg/kg.
    (D) 1 mg/kg.

68. You are treating a six-month-old infant who presents as "fussy." The infant is crying and has a respiratory rate of 40 per minute. She has pink skin with a capillary refill of 2 seconds. The cardiac monitor shows a narrow complex tachycardia of 260 beats per minute. Based on this assessment, the correct pharmacological intervention to control the rate would be
    (A) adenosine 0.1 mg/kg IV.
    (B) amiodarone 5 mg/kg IV over 20 minutes.
    (C) procainamide 15 mg/kg IV over 30 minutes.
    (D) lidocaine 1 mg/kg IV bolus.

69. You are dispatched to a private residence for an eight-year-old boy complaining of trouble breathing. On arrival, you find the patient lethargic with blue lips and rapid labored respirations. He is able to answer questions with only one- or two-word sentences. Physical examination reveals a respiratory rate of 50 per minute; diminished breath sounds and crackles are heard over the right lung field with dullness to percussion. He also has a temperature of 104°F. Based on your assessment, this patient may be experiencing
    (A) cardiogenic shock.
    (B) a drug overdose.
    (C) respiratory distress.
    (D) respiratory failure, most probably due to pneumonia.

70. Following defibrillation of a 36-pound child with ventricular fibrillation, you should
    (A) assess for a central pulse.
    (B) defibrillate with 64 joules.
    (C) immediately resume CPR.
    (D) reassess the cardiac rhythm.

71. You are caring for a lethargic two-year-old. Her blood glucose test confirms hypoglycemia. You are able to establish IV access. What is the appropriate drug to administer?
    (A) 50% dextrose
    (B) 10 mg glucagon
    (C) Instant glucose
    (D) 25% dextrose

72. You are caring for a 13-year-old suffering from a tricyclic antidepressant overdose. What cardiac arrhythmia is likely to develop as a result of this type of overdose?
    (A) Tall, peaked T waves
    (B) SVT
    (C) Wide QRS complex and prolonged QT interval
    (D) Narrow QRS complexes with normal PR interval

73. While enjoying an "off" day from work, you hear your neighbor screaming. You rush outside to see her pulling her four-year-old child from the swimming pool. The child is limp, blue, and not responsive to any stimulus. What should you do?
    (A) Perform the Heimlich maneuver in an attempt to eliminate water from the lungs.
    (B) Begin chest compressions.
    (C) Send the mother to call 911; open the airway and initiate rescue breathing.
    (D) Go to your car and get your AED and attach it as soon as possible.

74. Defibrillation in an infant or child
    (A) is repeated every 2 minutes as indicated.
    (B) is indicated only for ventricular fibrillation.
    (C) should be limited to one shock every 5 minutes.
    (D) requires an initial energy setting of 4 joules/kg.

75. You are called to the scene of a two-year-old child with a three-day history of diarrhea. The child appears to be in no respiratory distress with good breath sounds bilaterally. The heart rate is 140 per minute and the BP is 86/60. Capillary refill is delayed at about four seconds. The peripheral pulses are weak. After obtaining vascular access, which of the following would be the next intervention?
    (A) Get a chest X-ray.
    (B) Initiate a dopamine infusion at 2–5 mcg/kg/minute.
    (C) Start oral hydration.
    (D) Administer a 20 cc/kg bolus of normal saline.

76. Which of the following clinical presentations is MOST consistent with cocaine ingestion in a child?
    (A) Diaphoresis, miosis, tachycardia, and bronchospasm
    (B) Hypertension, tachycardia, diaphoresis, and mydriasis
    (C) Miosis, bradycardia, hypoventilation, and hypotension
    (D) Mydriasis, diarrhea, hypothermia, and hallucinations

77. You have just delivered a full-term baby in the back of your ambulance. The initial APGAR score is 5. Treatment should consist of
    (A) CPR.
    (B) effective ventilation.
    (C) vascular access.
    (D) administration of epinephrine.

78. External signs that may indicate an intraabdominal injury in a pediatric patient may include
    (A) a contusion to the forehead, deformity of the right wrist.
    (B) pale skin, abdominal contusion, seat belt abrasions across the abdomen.
    (C) dilated pupils, bradycardia, poor peripheral pulses.
    (D) tracheal deviation, JVD.

79. Which of the following assessment finding would indicate that a pediatric patient is progressing from respiratory distress to respiratory failure?
    (A) Nasal flaring
    (B) Respiratory rate over 32
    (C) Poor muscle tone
    (D) Grunting/head bobbing

80. Identify the anatomical differences in the pediatric airway compared to the adult airway.
    (A) The airway diameter is larger, the larynx is more anterior, the tongue is proportionally smaller.
    (B) The airway diameter is larger, the larynx is more posterior, the tongue is proportionally smaller.
    (C) The airway diameter is smaller, the larynx is more anterior, the tongue is proportionally larger.
    (D) The airway diameter is smaller, the larynx is more posterior, the tongue is proportionally larger.

81. Beta blocker ingestion in small children would MOST likely cause
    (A) acute hypoglycemia.
    (B) agitation or irritability.
    (C) marked hypertension.
    (D) ventricular fibrillation.

82. It is important to compare central and peripheral pulses in the pediatric patient to determine
    (A) the presence of shock.
    (B) skin color.
    (C) mental status.
    (D) airway patency.

83. A child wearing a helmet strikes a large rock on his bicycle and flies over the handlebars. The patient would MOST likely suffer
    (A) associated head injury.
    (B) stretching or tearing injuries to the kidneys.
    (C) open or closed fractures of the lower extremities.
    (D) compression injuries to the intraabdominal organs.

84. Of the following choices below, which is most likely to result from shaken baby syndrome?
    (A) Hypoglycemia
    (B) Abdominal bruising
    (C) Subdural hematoma
    (D) Lower extremity fracture

85. You have administered _____ to an eight-year-old. Drowsiness, decreased mental status, muscle twitching, and seizures are side effects that may result from its administration.
    (A) atropine
    (B) lidocaine
    (C) calcium chloride
    (D) adenosine

86. Your squad is dispatched to the scene of a six-year-old child with an elevated temperature. The mother tells you that the child was fine last night and got up this morning complaining of a sore throat and trouble swallowing. The initial assessment reveals a sick-looking child who is leaning forward in the tripod position. He is obviously drooling. From this information, you suspect
    (A) bronchiolitis.
    (B) croup.
    (C) epiglottitis.
    (D) meningitis.

87. During transport of a child with epiglottitis, he becomes unresponsive and apneic. You are still able to palpate a weak pulse at a rate of 64 per minute. Your immediate action should be to
    (A) apply a nonrebreather mask with 10–15 liters per minute of oxygen.
    (B) insert an OPA and administer bag-valve mask ventilations.
    (C) position the child's head and provide bag-valve mask ventilation with 100% oxygen.
    (D) immediately intubate the child.

88. Your patient is an ill-appearing four-month-old lying in his mother's arms. The mother tells you that the infant won't take a bottle and cries whenever he moves. Your exam reveals a lethargic infant, warm to touch, with fine pinpoint petechia on the abdomen, chest, and face. The infant's fontanelle appears to be bulging. The information gained on exam should lead you to suspect
    (A) bronchiolitis.
    (B) meningitis.
    (C) croup.
    (D) epiglottitis.

89. Select the statement that correctly relates to pediatric seizures.
    (A) Febrile seizures correlate to the speed in which the temperature rises, not to the degree of the fever.
    (B) Always suspect a fever to be the cause of a seizure if the temperature is more than 101°F.
    (C) Infants and children between the ages of four months and eight years commonly suffer from febrile seizures.
    (D) Febrile seizures do not require transport if the patient can be cooled.

Questions 90–92 are based on the following scenario:
You are dispatched to a local department store when a concerned customer notices an infant left unattended in a car. It is bitterly cold outside. Once you gain entry into the car, you find the infant to be dusky in color with no activity or movement. The respiratory rate is 12 per minute and irregular with grunting and short sighs. The heart rate is 64 per minute with weak central pulses. The infant's hands and feet are cold to touch. Capillary refill is 5 seconds.

90. Your immediate action would be to
    (A) start CPR.
    (B) ventilate with a bag-valve mask device and 100% oxygen.
    (C) give oxygen by blow-by.
    (D) intubate the infant.

91. After the above treatment is given, the infant does not improve. The ECG shows narrow complexes with P waves. The rate is 64 per minute. Your next action would be to obtain IV access and give
    (A) atropine for the bradycardia.
    (B) atropine 0.01–0.02 mg/kg.
    (C) 0.01 mg/kg of 1:1,000 epinephrine.
    (D) 0.01 mg/kg of 1:10,000 epinephrine.

92. After obtaining venous access and delivering the pharmacological intervention, the patient's heart rate increases to 130 per minute with strong central pulses but no peripheral pulses. To further stabilize the infant, the next course of action should be to
    (A) repeat the atropine dose.
    (B) repeat the epinephrine dose.
    (C) continue CPR.
    (D) begin rewarming the patient.

---

93. A seven-year-old child has been struck by a car and is lying motionless in the street. He has obvious head trauma. Identify the signs of Cushing's triad.

    (A) Increased BP, bradycardia, abnormal respirations
    (B) Decreased BP, tachycardia, increased respirations
    (C) Increased BP, tachycardia, increased respirations
    (D) Decreased BP, bradycardia, abnormal respirations

94. From the following list, identify an example of distributive shock.
    (A) Hypovolemic shock
    (B) Anaphylactic shock
    (C) Cardiogenic shock
    (D) Psychogenic shock

95. Seizurelike activity triggered by stimuli other than cerebral electrical discharges, such as major mood disorders or severe environmental stress, is defined as
    (A) partial seizure.
    (B) partial complex seizure.
    (C) generalized seizure.
    (D) pseudoseizure.

96. You are caring for a child with respiratory distress. You note a harsh high-pitched sound with each breath. You suspect this is indicative of
    (A) stridor.
    (B) wheezing.
    (C) crackles.
    (D) rhonchi.

97. Which of the following vital signs is most likely present in a 13-year-old with spinal shock?
    (A) BP 64/30; pulse 56 per minute
    (B) BP 64/30; pulse 150 per minute
    (C) BP 160/100; pulse 56 per minute
    (D) BP 160/100; pulse 150 per minute

98. To ensure that an infant's head is in a neutral position during spinal immobilization, you should
    (A) provide slight flexion of the head.
    (B) place padding under the infant's shoulders.
    (C) place a towel roll behind the infant's neck.
    (D) use towel rolls for lateral head stabilization.

99. You respond to a MVC involving a young child. The child is found apneic but still has a palpable pulse. You immediately begin positive pressure ventilation with a bag-valve mask device. You note that the left side of the chest moves, but the right does not. Lung sounds are absent on the right side and the trachea is deviated to the left. Your immediate action is to
    (A) increase the tidal volume with each ventilation.
    (B) perform a needle decompression on the left side.
    (C) give a 20 cc/kg bolus of IV fluids.
    (D) perform a needle decompression on the right side.

100. A 12-year-old, 40-pound child is experiencing an acute asthma attack that has been unresponsive to four puffs of an albuterol inhaler. The patient is conscious and alert but is notably dyspneic and has diffuse wheezing. Treatment includes
    (A) giving 0.35 mg of epinephrine 1:1,000 SQ.
    (B) giving 0.5 mg of nebulized ipratropium.
    (C) administer another 2.5-mg dose of albuterol.
    (D) assist ventilations with a bag-mask device.

101. Your assessment of an unresponsive 7-year-old, 60-pound child reveals that he is apneic and pulseless. After performing a 2-minute period of CPR, you assess his cardiac rhythm, which reveals ventricular fibrillation. You should
    (A) continue high-quality CPR and reassess in 2 minutes.
    (B) defibrillate and immediately resume CPR.
    (C) start an IV and administer epinephrine 1:10,000.
    (D) charge the defibrillator to 80 joules while CPR is ongoing.

102. A small child has fallen through the ice while skating. After 30 minutes, the child is pulled from the icy water apneic and pulseless. Your first action in the management of this child should be to
    (A) keep the child cool to maintain the mammalian dive reflex.
    (B) defibrillate the child immediately.
    (C) pronounce the child dead at the scene.
    (D) secure the child's airway and control the cervical spine.

103. You have intubated a six-week-old infant found in respiratory arrest. While performing ventilations, the child becomes blue and the pulse rate drops into the lower 50s. Your next step should be to
    (A) check the pulse oximeter reading.
    (B) administer epinephrine down the endotracheal tube to correct the bradycardia.
    (C) auscultate the chest.
    (D) administer atropine.

104. A child has suffered multisystem trauma and IV access cannot be obtained. You determine the best course of action would be to establish an IO. A contraindication for IO insertion is
    (A) a child is under one year old.
    (B) a child who is apneic and pulseless.
    (C) a fracture of the lower extremity.
    (D) a previous attempt in the opposite leg.

105. An injury to which abdominal organ is most likely to cause death in the pediatric patient?
     (A) Pancreas
     (B) Liver
     (C) Spleen
     (D) Kidney

106. You have performed a Rapid Trauma Survey on a child and are prepared to transport. In which situation is it appropriate to perform the detailed exam enroute to the hospital?
     (A) Fracture of the humerus
     (B) Amputated thumb
     (C) Mottled skin with tachycardia
     (D) Fractured tibia with numbness in the foot

107. You are treating a child with a tension pneumothorax. Needle decompression is needed. The correct site for insertion of the needle is
     (A) below the third rib in the midclavicular line.
     (B) below the second rib in the midaxillary line.
     (C) top of the second rib in the midaxillary line.
     (D) top of the third rib in the midclavicular line.

108. Of the statements below, identify that which is true concerning pediatric airway management.
     (A) The Sellick maneuver is not appropriate for use in the child.
     (B) Nasotracheal intubation is the preferred method of intubation.
     (C) Cuffed endotracheal tubes can be used in children.
     (D) Bradycardia can result from suctioning a child.

109. Which of the following is most likely to cause shock in a child?
     (A) Laceration to the face
     (B) A fractured radius
     (C) Cerebral edema
     (D) A splenic injury

110. Which action is most important when treating an unresponsive child?
     (A) Performing chest compressions
     (B) Checking for a pulse
     (C) Administering supplemental oxygen
     (D) Manually opening the airway

111. The minimum chest compression rate for a two-year-old in cardiac arrest is
    (A) 80/minute.
    (B) 100/minute.
    (C) 110/minute.
    (D) 120/minute.

112. The compression-ventilation ratio for two-rescuer CPR in an infant in cardiac arrest is
    (A) 5:1.
    (B) 3:1.
    (C) 15:2.
    (D) 5:2.

113. What is the first pharmacological agent to be administered in a pediatric cardiac arrest?
    (A) Atropine 1.0 mg
    (B) Epinephrine 1:10,000
    (C) Lidocaine 1 mg/kg
    (D) Epinephrine 1:1,000

114. In a pediatric patient, initial defibrillation should be performed at
    (A) 0.5 J/kg.
    (B) 4 J/kg.
    (C) 2 J/kg.
    (D) 100 J.

115. In a pediatric patient, initial cardioversion should be performed at
    (A) 0.5–1.0 J/kg.
    (B) 4 J/kg.
    (C) 2 J/kg.
    (D) 100 J.

116. You need to administer diazepam for a three-year-old in status epilepticus. He weighs 15 kg. An acceptable dose range is
    (A) 1.5–4.5 mg.
    (B) 1.0–3.5 mg.
    (C) 2.0–5 mg.
    (D) 0.01 mg/kg.

117. In caring for an infant burn patient, the rule of nines assigns _____ percent of the body surface area to the head.
    (A) 9%
    (B) 4½%
    (C) 18%
    (D) 36%

118. You respond to the local high school football practice field for a sports injury. The coach tells you that the patient made a tackle and after the play did not get up. Your patient is supine on the ground with all of his equipment on. He is awake but slow to answer questions. You should remove the football helmet if
    (A) a c-spine injury is suspected.
    (B) you do not have easy access to the airway.
    (C) you suspect the patient had a loss of consciousness.
    (D) the patient has numbness in his hands.

119. A priority in evaluating a two-year-old with diarrhea and vomiting includes determining
    (A) temperature elevation.
    (B) a viral infection.
    (C) a respiratory infection.
    (D) adequate hydration.

120. Cuffed endotracheal tubes are usually not indicated in children under what age?
    (A) Five
    (B) Eight
    (C) Three
    (D) Ten

ANSWERS AND ANSWER EXPLANATIONS

1. **(B)** Supine hypotension syndrome (or vena cava syndrome) occurs when the pregnant uterus compresses the inferior vena cava when the patient is in a supine position. This results in a decrease in blood return back to the heart and a reduction of cardiac output. This syndrome can occur as early as the third month of gestation.

2. **(A)** The backboard must be tilted on its left side 10–15 degrees to prevent supine hypotension syndrome. Tilting the board will allow the uterus to displace to the left and prevent compression of the inferior vena cava.

3. **(C)** The major concern with a prolapsed cord is compression of the cord by the head of the infant. This can result in a reduced blood flow to the infant and lead to fetal hypoxia.

4. **(C)** Mittelschmerz is German for "middle pain" and is defined as abdominal pain in the region of the ovary during ovulation.

5. **(B)** Parity refers to the number of viable deliveries. This is common obstetric medical terminology you must be familiar with.

6. **(A)** Abruptio placenta is premature separation of the placenta from the uterus. There are different presentations that can occur depending on the severity of the abruption. Classic presentation includes a sudden, sharp, tearing pain and the development of a stiff boardlike abdomen. Bleeding can be severe or not present depending on many factors.

7. **(C)** Abruptio placenta is premature separation of the placenta from the uterus and is a true medical emergency because it poses a life threat to the mother and fetus.

8. **(D)** Multigravida is when a woman has been pregnant more than once. Nullipara is a woman who has not yet delivered her first child. If you did not know this common terminology, you must review obstetric medical terminology.

9. **(C)** Normal physiological changes to vital signs during the second trimester of pregnancy include a drop in blood pressure 10–15 mmHg due to a reduction in peripheral vascular resistance. The heart rate will increase 10–20 beats per minute due to an increased maternal blood volume. Note: The blood pressure will rise back to baseline in the third trimester.

10. **(D)** Common signs and symptoms of preeclampsia include headache, dizziness, confusion, blurred vision, nausea, vomiting, proteinuria, hypertension, and edema.

11. **(D)** Position the mother with the hips elevated as much as possible or in the knee-chest position in an attempt to relieve pressure on the cord.

12. **(B)** You would instruct the patient to pant with each contraction to prevent bearing down and applying pressure on the cord.

13. **(C)** With a gloved hand, place two fingers into the vagina to elevate the presenting part to relieve pressure on the cord. Provide oxygen and rapid transport to a hospital that can perform a cesarean delivery.

14. **(A)** Applying a sterile dressing to the exposed cord will minimize temperature change. If the cord is exposed to room temperature, the temperature of blood flowing to the infant will decrease. This can cause hypothermia. Additionally, a temperature change of the blood may cause the umbilical vessels to spasm resulting in decreased blood flow to the infant.

15. **(D)** Oxytocin is a hormone secreted by the pituitary gland that stimulates the uterus to produce stronger contractions. The medication Pitocin (oxytocin) is used to induce labor or control postpartum hemorrhage.

16. **(A)** Chlamydia trachomatis is the most common sexually transmitted disease in the United States. Gonorrhea, syphilis, and herpesvirus are also sexually transmitted diseases.

17. **(B)** Pelvic inflammatory disease is often accompanied by increased pain when walking. The patient will bend forward and take short, slow steps. Guarding of the abdomen and nausea are also common with PID.

18. **(B)** Common signs and symptoms of preeclampsia include headache, dizziness, confusion, blurred vision, nausea, vomiting, proteinuria, hypertension, and edema.

19. **(D)** If you suspect preeclampsia, you should take precautions to prevent seizures, which include keeping the patient calm, and transporting without lights and sirens.

20. **(C)** Treatment of seizure activity in eclampsia includes placing the patient in the left lateral recumbent position, maintaining the airway, administering high-flow oxygen, establishing IV access, and the administration of 2–5 grams of magnesium sulfate IV. If seizures cannot be controlled, sedatives may be required.

21. **(B)** Placenta previa is usually in a multigravida in her third trimester of pregnancy. A recent history of sexual intercourse or vaginal examination just before the onset of vaginal bleeding is not uncommon. The onset of painless bright red vaginal bleeding or spotting is considered the hallmark sign of placenta previa.

22. **(C)** A vaginal exam should not be attempted when placenta previa is suspected. The exam may puncture the placenta and cause a severe hemorrhage.

23. **(B)** It is important to wait one full minute to perform the first APGAR assessment. A second APGAR should be performed at five minutes.

24. **(C)** If the amniotic sac is present around the baby's head, use your fingers to pinch the sac and then push it away from the nose and mouth. Using a scalpel or scissors is *not* recommended.

25. **(D)** This is one of the most basic OB questions you can be asked. If you missed this question, you need to review childbirth.

26. **(A)** If a newborn's heart rate is 60–80 and does not increase despite stimulation and ventilation, it is necessary to start chest compressions.

27. **(B)** An ectopic pregnancy should be suspected when abdominal pain is present in women of childbearing age who are sexually active. An ectopic pregnancy can be difficult to distinguish from other conditions. The classic triad of symptoms includes abdominal pain, vaginal bleeding, and amenorrhea. Other symptoms include referred pain to the shoulder, nausea, vomiting, or syncope. Signs of shock may be present if the ectopic ruptures.

28. **(C)** The placenta has many functions including the transport of oxygen, nutrients, and other substances to the fetus and the excretion of CO_2 and other waste products. Production of hormones is not a function of the placenta.

29. **(A)** EMS providers should limit the patient's history to the elements necessary to provide care. Patient contact should be nonjudgmental and supportive.

30. **(B)** Gravida or gravidity refers to the number of times a woman has been pregnant. If you did not know this common terminology, you must review obstetric medical terminology.

31. **(B)** Preparation for delivery is necessary. The information presented in this scenario should lead you to believe that delivery of the baby is imminent.

32. **(C)** This is a trauma patient who requires 100% oxygen, rapid extrication from the vehicle with c-spine immobilization onto a backboard, placing the backboard on the left side (to prevent supine hypotension syndrome), and establishing two large-bore IVs while enroute to the hospital.

33. **(B)** Treatment for a pregnant patient in cardiac arrest would include defibrillation, CPR, intubation, and administration of appropriate medications.

34. **(A)** An ectopic pregnancy should be suspected when abdominal pain is present in women of childbearing age who are sexually active, an ectopic pregnancy can be difficult to distinguish from other conditions. The classic triad of symptoms includes abdominal pain, vaginal bleeding, and amenorrhea. Other symptoms include referred pain to the shoulder, nausea, vomiting, or syncope. Signs of shock may be present if the ectopic ruptures.

35. **(C)** If central cyanosis is present, or you are unsure about the adequacy of ventilation, the administration of supplemental oxygen is necessary. Never deprive a newborn of oxygen for fear of oxygen toxicity.

36. **(A)** Keep the newborn at the same level of the vagina with the head slightly lower than the rest of the body. This will prevent over- or undertransfusion of blood from the umbilical cord to the newborn and facilitate drainage of secretions from the nose and mouth to help prevent aspiration.

37. **(B)** The umbilical cord consists of one vein and two arteries. The umbilical vein carries oxygenated blood from the placenta to the fetus. The umbilical arteries transport waste products from the fetus to the placenta.

38. **(A)** The Leopold maneuver is palpation of the abdomen in four different assessment steps. This is used to identify the number of fetuses, the fetal presentation, presenting part, degree of descent, point of maximum intensity of fetal heart tones, and internal rotation of the fetus.

39. **(C)** Contraction intervals are correctly measured from the beginning of one contraction to the beginning of the next. Many health care providers incorrectly measure intervals from the end of one contraction to the beginning of the next.

40. **(A)** Contraction length is correctly measured from the beginning of the contraction to the end of that contraction.

41. **(B)** Regular contractions lasting 45–60 seconds at one- to two-minute intervals and crowning indicate delivery is imminent.

42. **(B)** Initial care for nuchal cord (cord around the neck) is to first try to gently remove the cord from around the neck. If this is not successful and the cord is so tight that it is inhibiting labor, it will be necessary to clamp the cord in two places and cut between the clamps.

43. **(C)** If the infant starts to breathe with its face pressed against the vaginal wall, it is necessary to insert two fingers in the vagina to form an airway around the infant's nose and mouth.

44. **(C)** Applying gentle countertraction to the infant's head to prevent explosive delivery is essential to decrease the likelihood of tearing of the perineum and decreases the potential for rapid expulsion of the baby's skull through the birth canal, which may cause intracranial injury.

45. **(A)** Meconium-stained amniotic fluid indicates a fetal hypoxic incident. Hypoxia causes an increase in digestive activity along with the relaxation of the anal sphincter, which allows meconium to pass into the amniotic fluid.

46. **(B)** Croup is a viral infection of the upper airway that causes inflammation of the subglottic region that can lead to airway obstruction. Inspiratory stridor is often present. Other assessment findings include nasal flaring, tracheal tugging or retractions. The vital signs of this patient are compensatory to the airway obstruction.

47. **(D)** Respiratory failure is evident for the following reasons: tachypnea, tachycardia, nasal flaring, retractions, audible airway noises (stridor/barky) cough, and slowness to respond, which indicates a decreased level of consciousness.

48. **(B)** The child is unstable (decreased LOC, rapid heart rate, and hypotension). Synchronized cardioversion should be provided at 0.5–1.0 joule per kilogram.

49. **(D)** Naloxone is used to reverse the effects of opiate toxicity. The recommended dose in pediatrics is 0.1 mg/kg.

50. **(C)** Fluid resuscitation for multisystem trauma in the pediatric patient includes a bolus of an isotonic crystalloid at 20 cc/kg. Reassess and repeat as needed.

51. **(A)** Respiratory distress is defined as the inability to maintain gaseous exchange sufficient to meet the needs of the body. Evidence of abnormal respirations (tachypnea or bradypnea) or increased work of breathing; use of accessory muscles, nasal flaring, grunting, and decreased mentation can also signal respiratory distress in the pediatric patient.

52. **(D)** A length-based resuscitation tape should be used to help determine proper endotracheal tube size. If one is not available, the following formula can be used: (age + 16) ÷ 4 = size of tube (in mm).

53. **(B)** The result of violent shaking in a baby less that 24 months old may include damage to nerve tissues deep within the brain and torn veins between the brain and the skull, which can cause severe bleeding.

54. (A) You may suspect shaken baby syndrome based on bulging of the anterior fontanelle without fever or overhydration as a cause. In addition, the multiple areas of bruising provide information that may indicate child abuse.

55. (C) Characteristics of a newborn with fetal alcohol syndrome include low birth weight, a small head, and small eye openings.

56. (D) Inspiratory stridor, absence of drooling, trouble swallowing, and symptoms persistently worse at night leads to the conclusion of the croup.

57. (B) IO infusions will generally improve the patient's condition or improve his or her vascular volume, thereby increasing the BP and cardiac output. Osteomyelitis (A) can occur if the needle is left in place for longer than 24 hours; fractures (C) can occur when the extremity is not well stabilized or an attempt was made at a improper site where the bone is weaker; compartment syndrome (D) occurs when extravasation is not detected.

58. (B) 0.01 mg/kg IV/IO of 1:10,000 solution is the recommended dose of epinephrine for pediatric cardiac arrest and/or symptoms of bradycardia.

59. (D) 5 mg/kg of amiodarone is the recommended dose for the treatment of pulseless v tach or v fib in a pediatric patient.

60. (D) A length-based resuscitation tape should be used to help determine proper orogastric tube size. If one is not available, determine the proper endotracheal tube size using the following formula: (age + 16) ÷ 4 = size of tube (in mm). The proper orogastric tube size will be double the ET tube size. For example, a child requiring a 5.0 mm ET tube will require a 10F orogastric tube.

61. (B) 15 compressions to 2 ventilations is the proper compression/ventilation ratio for two-rescuer CPR.

62. (C) Heart rates ranging from 180 to 220 beats per minute in a child is considered SVT if the QRS complexes remain narrow. V tach (A) presents with a wide QRS; sinus tachycardia (D) usually shows waves and, rapid atrial fibrillation (B) will be irregularly irregular.

63. (D) Epinephrine is the drug of choice for symptomatic bradycardia in the pediatric patient. Atropine (A) is effective in the *adult* bradycardic patient since bradycardia is often a result of parasympathetic stimulation; lidocaine (B) is contraindicated in bradycardia. (C) is not indicated.

64. **(C)** Allowing the chest to recoil fully between compressions is a key component in the revised American Heart Association guidelines.

65. **(B)** Applying ice to the face of the infant, being careful not to obstruct the nose and mouth. If the child is old enough to follow directions, have the child hold his/her breath and blow into an occluded straw or encourage the child to bear down.

66. **(A)** Amiodarone is the drug of choice for stable wide complex tachycardia in children.

67. **(D)** The pediatric dose of lidocaine is 1 mg/kg bolus given IV/IO in cardiac arrest with a presenting rhythm of ventricular fibrillation or pulseless ventricular tachycardia.

68. **(A)** In a pediatric patient, adenosine given at 0.1 mg/kg IV is indicated to correct a stable tachycardia.

69. **(D)** The patient may be experiencing respiratory failure, most probably due to pneumonia based on tachypnea, increased work of breathing, diminished breath sounds, dullness to percussions, and elevated temperature.

70. **(C)** CPR should be resumed following defibrillation. After 5 cycles of CPR, reassess the rhythm and pulse and defibrillate again if a shockable rhythm is present.

71. **(D)** A 25% dextrose solution is recommended for pediatric patients because it is less viscous than 50% dextrose. This will allow easier administration through a smaller diameter IV catheter and reduce the occurrence of sclerosis to small peripheral veins.

72. **(C)** TCA overdose produces a prolonged QT interval along with widening of the QRS complex. Tall, peaked T waves are most commonly associated with hyperkalemia.

73. **(C)** The lone rescuer should initially provide rescue breathing to the child while someone is sent to call 911.

74. **(A)** After 5 cycles of CPR (2 minutes), reassess the rhythm and pulse and defibrillate again if a shockable rhythm is present.

75. **(D)** With the vital signs given in the scenario, the child is displaying signs and symptoms consistent with compensated shock. The shock is most probably related to diarrhea. A 20 cc/kg bolus of normal saline or an isotonic crystalloid fluid is recommended.

76. **(B)** Hypertension, tachycardia, diaphoresis, and mydriasis (dilated pupils) are consistent with cocaine or amphetamine use.

77. **(B)** Most newborn infants respond quite favorably to warming, drying, suctioning, and stimulation. Occasionally, administration of oxygen with assisted ventilations may be necessary. Vascular access and CPR are utilized only after the infant fails to respond effectively to ventilatory assistance.

78. **(B)** Pale skin, abdominal contusion, seat belt abrasions, or unexplained shock may suggest the possibility of intraabdominal injury with a probability of abdominal hemorrhage.

79. **(C)** Nasal flaring, elevated respiratory rate, grunting, and head bobbing all indicate respiratory distress. The development of poor muscle tone indicates the patient is tiring and is an ominous sign of respiratory failure.

80. **(C)** The airway diameter in children is smaller than an adult airway; the larynx is more anterior making visualization difficult; the tongue is proportionally larger to the jaw.

81. **(A)** Ingestion of beta blockers, ethanol or other alcohols, insulin, or oral hypoglycemic agents can lead to hypoglycemia.

82. **(A)** The presence or absence of shock may be indicated by a difference between the central and peripheral pulses. Pulse differences or deficit may be a sign of poor peripheral perfusion.

83. **(D)** Injury from bicycle handlebars typically includes compression injuries to the intraabdominal organs and pancreatic injuries. Upper extremity injuries are also common.

84. **(C)** Head injury (including the possibility of a subdural hematoma) is a common finding in shaken baby syndrome.

85. **(B)** Lidocaine has central nervous system properties that cause drowsiness, decreased mental status, muscle twitching, and the possibility of seizures.

86. **(C)** Epiglottitis is a bacterial infection causing the acute swelling of the epiglottis and the soft tissues above the glottic opening. Clinical findings include but are not limited to sudden onset high fever (102–105°F), pain on swallowing, typically sitting in tripod position, and drooling.

87. **(C)** Any external manipulation of the epiglottis (i.e., intubation or OPA insertion) can cause complete airway obstruction in the child with epiglottitis. Carefully position the child's head and provide positive pressure ventilation with 100% oxygen.

88. **(B)** Recognize the syndrome of fever and petechia as a medical emergency. Inflammation of the meninges will cause the fontanelle to bulge and appear full. Meningitis should be suspected in this patient.

89. **(A)** How fast the temperature of the child rises will increase a child's risk for developing a seizure. For example, a child who transitions from a temperature of 100.2 to 104.5°F in 30 minutes is more likely to suffer a febrile seizure than a child who develops a 104.5°F temperature over several hours.

90. **(B)** Recognize that the infant has inadequate oxygenation (dusky color) and immediately begin bag-valve mask ventilation with 100% oxygen.

91. **(D)** Epinephrine 1:10,000 solution should be given at 0.01 mg/kg IV/IO for persistent bradycardia unresponsive to ventilation.

92. **(D)** Considering the ambient temperature to be very cold in this scenario, hypothermia is a significant cause of the patient's presentation. Begin rewarming the patient.

93. **(A)** Cushing's triad (sometimes referred to as Cushing's reflex or response) characteristically presents with an elevated blood pressure, bradycardia, and abnormal (usually slow) respirations.

94. **(B)** Distributive shock is a shock state that exists when there is no loss of body fluid, but the fluid distribution is altered from an increase in the vascular space or leaking of fluid from the vascular space. This results in an insufficiency of fluid relative to the vascular space. Types of distributive shock include anaphylactic, septic, and neurogenic.

95. **(D)** Pseudoseizures are triggered by any mechanism other than cerebral electrical discharge.

96. **(A)** Stridor is a harsh high or low-pitched sound caused by breathing through a partially blocked airway; wheezing **(B)** is a high or low-pitched whistling sound; crackles/rhonchi **(C)** and **(D)** represent fluid in the larger bronchial airways.

97. **(A)** Spinal shock (neurogenic) is a distributive shock producing hypotension relative to an increase in the vascular space in the absence of a loss of body fluids. A spinal cord injury results in a "lack of communication" between the brain and the body so there is no response to catecholamine release resulting in bradycardia and hypotension.

98. **(B)** An infant has a large head in comparison to the rest of the body. To maintain the infant's head in a neutral position, place padding under the infant's shoulders.

99. **(D)** The signs and symptoms are consistent with a tension pneumothorax (absent breath sounds, tracheal deviation, no or little chest movement on the affected side). Immediate needle decompression is warranted.

100. **(B)** Children with moderate respiratory distress may benefit from inhaled ipratropium. A combination of ipratropium and albuterol is more effective than albuterol alone.

101. **(B)** After 5 cycles of CPR (2 minutes), reassess the rhythm and pulse and defibrillate again if a shockable rhythm is present.

102. **(D)** Since it is unknown if there are any c-spine injuries from the fall through the ice, you must secure the airway and control the cervical spine during resuscitation.

103. **(C)** Auscultation of the chest for proper endotracheal tube placement is necessary. If lung sounds are diminished or absent, it may be necessary to extubate, ventilate, reassess, and then reintubate.

104. **(C)** A fracture of the lower extremity is a contraindication to an IO insertion.

105. **(B)** The liver is a solid, vascular organ in the right upper quadrant. Rupture or laceration of the liver can cause severe hemorrhage. Injury to the liver is the most common abdominal injury that leads to death in the pediatric patient.

106. **(C)** A sign of poor perfusion includes mottled skin and tachycardia. This is indicative of shock and a detailed exam should be performed enroute to the hospital. Other indicators of shock include weak peripheral pulses and prolonged capillary refill time.

107. **(D)** Inserting the needle over (on top of) the second or third rib avoids inadvertent puncturing or laceration of the adjoining vessels and nerves located at the inferior border of the ribs.

108. **(D)** Suctioning may result in bradycardia from stimulation of the vagus nerve, particularly in children less than six months old. Do not use prolonged suction attempts.

109. **(D)** The spleen is a blood-filled organ located in the left upper quadrant. Blunt trauma can cause injury to the spleen resulting in blood loss and shock. The spleen is the most injured organ resulting in *shock,* while the liver is the most injured organ resulting in *death* of a pediatric patient.

110. **(D)** Establishing a patent airway is the most important treatment step in providing care for an unresponsive patient. This is basic life support material you must be familiar with before taking your certification exam.

111. **(B)** The answer is a minimum of 100 chest compressions per minute. This is basic life support material you must be familiar with before taking your certification exam.

112. **(C)** Fifteen compressions to two ventilations. This is basic life support material you must be familiar with before taking your certification exam.

113. **(B)** Epinephrine 0.01 mg/kg of 1:10,000 solution is the recommended dose for pediatric cardiac arrest and/or symptoms of bradycardia.

114. **(C)** The recommended energy setting when defibrillation is necessary is 2 joules/kg. Repeat defibrillation is recommended at 4 joules/kg.

115. **(A)** The recommended energy setting when cardioversion is necessary is 0.5–1.0 joules/kg. Repeat cardioversion can be increased to 2 joules/kg.

116. **(A)** The dose range for diazepam is 0.1–0.3 mg/kg. A 15 kg patient would receive 1.5 to 4.5 mg of medication.

117. **(C)** Using the rule of nines, the head of an infant is assigned 18% body surface area.

118. **(B)** Unless special circumstances exist such as respiratory distress or airway compromise, the helmet should not be removed by EMS. This question asks when you *should* remove the helmet. Not having easy access to the airway is the best choice.

119. **(D)** Of the choices listed, evaluating the patient for adequate hydration is the top priority. Evaluating the patient's temperature **(A)** and the presence of infection **(B)** and **(C)** are necessary but secondary to determining adequate hydration.

120. **(B)** Cuffed endotracheal tubes are not indicated for children under the age of eight. In a child less than eight, the normal anatomic narrowing at the level of the cricoid cartilage provides a "functional cuff," and eliminates the need for a cuffed tracheal tube under most circumstances.

Notes

Operations

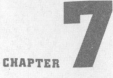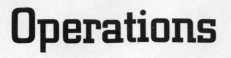

This chapter covers a variety of topics including scene safety, legal considerations, vehicle operations, communications, documentation, infection control, quality improvement, DNR, basic patient assessment, basic physiology, hazardous materials, mass casualty incidents, and scene management.

Answer Sheet
CHAPTER 7—OPERATIONS

1 Ⓐ Ⓑ Ⓒ Ⓓ	21 Ⓐ Ⓑ Ⓒ Ⓓ	41 Ⓐ Ⓑ Ⓒ Ⓓ	61 Ⓐ Ⓑ Ⓒ Ⓓ
2 Ⓐ Ⓑ Ⓒ Ⓓ	22 Ⓐ Ⓑ Ⓒ Ⓓ	42 Ⓐ Ⓑ Ⓒ Ⓓ	62 Ⓐ Ⓑ Ⓒ Ⓓ
3 Ⓐ Ⓑ Ⓒ Ⓓ	23 Ⓐ Ⓑ Ⓒ Ⓓ	43 Ⓐ Ⓑ Ⓒ Ⓓ	63 Ⓐ Ⓑ Ⓒ Ⓓ
4 Ⓐ Ⓑ Ⓒ Ⓓ	24 Ⓐ Ⓑ Ⓒ Ⓓ	44 Ⓐ Ⓑ Ⓒ Ⓓ	64 Ⓐ Ⓑ Ⓒ Ⓓ
5 Ⓐ Ⓑ Ⓒ Ⓓ	25 Ⓐ Ⓑ Ⓒ Ⓓ	45 Ⓐ Ⓑ Ⓒ Ⓓ	65 Ⓐ Ⓑ Ⓒ Ⓓ
6 Ⓐ Ⓑ Ⓒ Ⓓ	26 Ⓐ Ⓑ Ⓒ Ⓓ	46 Ⓐ Ⓑ Ⓒ Ⓓ	66 Ⓐ Ⓑ Ⓒ Ⓓ
7 Ⓐ Ⓑ Ⓒ Ⓓ	27 Ⓐ Ⓑ Ⓒ Ⓓ	47 Ⓐ Ⓑ Ⓒ Ⓓ	67 Ⓐ Ⓑ Ⓒ Ⓓ
8 Ⓐ Ⓑ Ⓒ Ⓓ	28 Ⓐ Ⓑ Ⓒ Ⓓ	48 Ⓐ Ⓑ Ⓒ Ⓓ	68 Ⓐ Ⓑ Ⓒ Ⓓ
9 Ⓐ Ⓑ Ⓒ Ⓓ	29 Ⓐ Ⓑ Ⓒ Ⓓ	49 Ⓐ Ⓑ Ⓒ Ⓓ	69 Ⓐ Ⓑ Ⓒ Ⓓ
10 Ⓐ Ⓑ Ⓒ Ⓓ	30 Ⓐ Ⓑ Ⓒ Ⓓ	50 Ⓐ Ⓑ Ⓒ Ⓓ	70 Ⓐ Ⓑ Ⓒ Ⓓ
11 Ⓐ Ⓑ Ⓒ Ⓓ	31 Ⓐ Ⓑ Ⓒ Ⓓ	51 Ⓐ Ⓑ Ⓒ Ⓓ	71 Ⓐ Ⓑ Ⓒ Ⓓ
12 Ⓐ Ⓑ Ⓒ Ⓓ	32 Ⓐ Ⓑ Ⓒ Ⓓ	52 Ⓐ Ⓑ Ⓒ Ⓓ	72 Ⓐ Ⓑ Ⓒ Ⓓ
13 Ⓐ Ⓑ Ⓒ Ⓓ	33 Ⓐ Ⓑ Ⓒ Ⓓ	53 Ⓐ Ⓑ Ⓒ Ⓓ	73 Ⓐ Ⓑ Ⓒ Ⓓ
14 Ⓐ Ⓑ Ⓒ Ⓓ	34 Ⓐ Ⓑ Ⓒ Ⓓ	54 Ⓐ Ⓑ Ⓒ Ⓓ	74 Ⓐ Ⓑ Ⓒ Ⓓ
15 Ⓐ Ⓑ Ⓒ Ⓓ	35 Ⓐ Ⓑ Ⓒ Ⓓ	55 Ⓐ Ⓑ Ⓒ Ⓓ	75 Ⓐ Ⓑ Ⓒ Ⓓ
16 Ⓐ Ⓑ Ⓒ Ⓓ	36 Ⓐ Ⓑ Ⓒ Ⓓ	56 Ⓐ Ⓑ Ⓒ Ⓓ	76 Ⓐ Ⓑ Ⓒ Ⓓ
17 Ⓐ Ⓑ Ⓒ Ⓓ	37 Ⓐ Ⓑ Ⓒ Ⓓ	57 Ⓐ Ⓑ Ⓒ Ⓓ	77 Ⓐ Ⓑ Ⓒ Ⓓ
18 Ⓐ Ⓑ Ⓒ Ⓓ	38 Ⓐ Ⓑ Ⓒ Ⓓ	58 Ⓐ Ⓑ Ⓒ Ⓓ	78 Ⓐ Ⓑ Ⓒ Ⓓ
19 Ⓐ Ⓑ Ⓒ Ⓓ	39 Ⓐ Ⓑ Ⓒ Ⓓ	59 Ⓐ Ⓑ Ⓒ Ⓓ	79 Ⓐ Ⓑ Ⓒ Ⓓ
20 Ⓐ Ⓑ Ⓒ Ⓓ	40 Ⓐ Ⓑ Ⓒ Ⓓ	60 Ⓐ Ⓑ Ⓒ Ⓓ	80 Ⓐ Ⓑ Ⓒ Ⓓ

1. A properly written patient care report (PCR) is important because
   (A) the PCR relays the paramedic's true opinion of the patient.
   (B) the PCR provides the receiving hospital with important billing information.
   (C) the PCR may be the only source for pertinent information for receiving healthcare professionals.
   (D) the PCR links traits of the paramedic with documentation abilities.

2. The PCR is a legal document making it necessary to record accurate
   (A) incident times.
   (B) paramedic certifications.
   (C) names of nearest relatives.
   (D) personal opinions.

3. Findings that require no medical intervention, but require documentation as evidence of a thorough history and exam are termed
   (A) negative responses.
   (B) positive therapeutics.
   (C) noteworthy responses.
   (D) pertinent negatives.

4. The proper way to correct a written error on the PCR is to
   (A) use White-Out to cover the error.
   (B) draw a single line through the error, initial, and date the area.
   (C) scribble through the error completely and sign your name next to the error.
   (D) use a black marker to eliminate the error from the PCR, initial, and date the area.

5. An incomplete or illegible patient care report
   (A) may be acceptable in some areas.
   (B) may cause subsequent caregivers to provide inappropriate treatment based on the report.
   (C) is of no use.
   (D) is useful in the ongoing care and treatment of the patient.

6. Documentation of a patient's refusal for care or transport should include all of the following except
   (A) the patient's insurance information.
   (B) the paramedic's advice to the patient.
   (C) online medical control's advice.
   (D) a complete narrative of the event.

7. Revisions to the original patient care report
   (A) should be added on the original document.
   (B) are never appropriate.
   (C) are done on a separate report form and then attached to the original.
   (D) can easily be done with a different color ink.

8. Appropriate professional language on a PCR includes
   (A) medical terminology.
   (B) slang.
   (C) personal opinion.
   (D) personally acceptable abbreviations.

9. A telephone is an example of a _____ communication system.
   (A) simplex
   (B) duplex
   (C) multiplex
   (D) trunked

10. For communication to be effective, the receiver must give appropriate _____ to the sender:
    (A) ideas
    (B) encodings
    (C) decodings
    (D) feedback

11. When communicating medical information, using proper terminology can
    (A) shorten transmission and provide an unambiguous form of communication.
    (B) serve no vital importance.
    (C) alter the interpretation of the nature of the incident if heard by several different people.
    (D) reflect upon the EMS professional negatively.

12. Disadvantages of a simplex system may include that
    (A) the process is slower and more formal.
    (B) either party can interrupt the other party as necessary.
    (C) voice transmission may interfere with data transmission.
    (D) simplex system facilitates discussion.

13. Disadvantages of using a cellular telephone for EMS communications include that
    (A) the conversation is less formal.
    (B) the system promotes discussion.
    (C) the system reduces online time.
    (D) geography can interfere with the system or signs.

14. The federal agency that regulates telecommunications in the United States
    is the
    (A) FBI.
    (B) FDIC.
    (C) FCC.
    (D) FACEP.

15. Functions of an EMS dispatcher include all of the following except
    (A) call taking.
    (B) proper diagnosis of the caller's illness.
    (C) alerting and directing the EMS response.
    (D) giving prearrival instructions to the caller.

16. Communication from the EMS dispatcher that provides the caller with
    emotional support, may be life sustaining to the patient during a critical
    event, provides immediate assistance to the caller as well as ongoing infor-
    mation to responding units is
    (A) incident data collection.
    (B) predispatch education.
    (C) prearrival instructions.
    (D) incident referral data.

17. Bacteria, viruses, and fungi are all examples of
    (A) pathogenetic hosts.
    (B) nonspecific inflammatory agents.
    (C) disease processes.
    (D) infectious agents.

18. The body's first line of defense against infection is
    (A) the skin.
    (B) the respiratory system.
    (C) the G.I. system.
    (D) humoral response.

19. You respond to the home of a patient with an unknown illness for two days.
    You approach the call suspecting an infectious or communicable disease.
    Which action is not appropriate for this patient's care?
    (A) Gloves and protective eye goggles are worn.
    (B) A full history and detailed physical exam is obtained.
    (C) Make the patient a "load and go" due to the potential for paramedic
        exposure.
    (D) Dispose of supplies and sharps appropriately on disposition of patient.

20. Proper care of the patient with known HIV includes all of the following except
    (A) isolation of the patient.
    (B) effective handwashing.
    (C) use of eye protection and gowns where exposure to bodily fluids in large quantities is possible.
    (D) BSI, based on task performed.

21. Of the following hepatitis groups, which is not transmitted via blood?
    (A) Hepatitis A
    (B) Hepatitis B
    (C) Hepatitis C
    (D) Hepatitis D

Questions 22 and 23 are based on the following scenario:

You are called to a local homeless shelter for a gentleman with complaint of a cough for two to three weeks, night sweats, and weight loss.

22. You suspect
    (A) hepatitis A.
    (B) HIV.
    (C) TB (tuberculosis).
    (D) meningitis.

23. You diagnose the above illness appropriately and know the disease is spread through
    (A) exposure to blood.
    (B) exposure through airborne droplets.
    (C) exposure to body fluids.
    (D) direct physical contact.

---

24. You respond to a home of a patient with complaint of sudden onset of fever/chills, joint pain, neck stiffness, and severe headache. Upon examination the medics note a petechial rash. You suspect

    (A) rabies.
    (B) influenza.
    (C) hepatitis A.
    (D) meningitis.

25. The causative organism of chicken pox is the varicella zoster virus, which is a member of the
    (A) varicella virus group.
    (B) zoster virus group.
    (C) herpesvirus group.
    (D) rubivirus group.

26. Reportable infectious/communicable disease exposures include
    (A) contact of infectious materials with eye, mouth, or mucous membrane.
    (B) working with a partner with a URI.
    (C) contact with blood and body fluids on intact gloves.
    (D) spill of infectious material in the EMS unit with no contact.

27. Legislation that governs the practice of medicine and may prescribe a physician's ability to delegate authority to perform medical acts by the paramedic is
    (A) licensure.
    (B) medical direction.
    (C) standard of care.
    (D) medical practice act.

28. Exercising the degree of care, skill, and judgment that would be expected under like or similar circumstances by a similarly trained, reasonable paramedic in a similar community or location is the definition of
    (A) duty to act.
    (B) standard of care.
    (C) malfeasance.
    (D) proximate cause.

29. The elements of a negligence claim include all of the following except
    (A) duty to act.
    (B) breach of duty.
    (C) code of conduct.
    (D) proximate cause.

30. You arrive on the scene of a two-car MVC. The driver of the first vehicle is unconscious. Consent for this patient is said to be
    (A) informed.
    (B) implied.
    (C) expressed.
    (D) involuntary.

31. You and your partner are treating a 16-year-old female with lower abdominal pain. The patient's husband arrives and informs you his wife may be pregnant. You can treat this patient without parental consent based on
    (A) the nonurgent doctrine.
    (B) an emancipated minor is considered an adult.
    (C) the fact that she is mentally competent.
    (D) the fact that the consent is involuntary.

32. You are called to the middle of a bridge to transport a violent patient who is suicidal. Per local police, the patient threatened to jump from the bridge and needs a psychiatric evaluation. The patient refuses transport threatening to sue anyone who touches him. You transport this patient against his will based on
    (A) informed consent.
    (B) implied consent.
    (C) expressed consent.
    (D) involuntary consent.

33. You and your partner are treating a patient who needs to be transported to the hospital for chest pain. You have established an IV, placed the patient on the monitor, administered oxygen and aspirin. Your partner checks his watch and notes that his shift is over. You remove the monitor and politely tell the patient the oncoming crew will come and transport him to the hospital shortly. Leaving this patient is an example of
    (A) false imprisonment.
    (B) assault.
    (C) battery.
    (D) abandonment.

34. Unlawful touching of an individual without his or her consent could leave the paramedic open to allegations of
    (A) assault.
    (B) battery.
    (C) abandonment.
    (D) false imprisonment.

35. Advance directives are documents that express the patient's wishes in the event that he or she is unconscious or otherwise unable to express his or her choice for care. These include living wills, do not resuscitate orders, and
    (A) slow code requests.
    (B) durable power of attorney for health care.
    (C) artificial care order.
    (D) health care denial form.

36. The paramedic's primary responsibility at a crime scene or accident scene is
    (A) quality patient care.
    (B) quality documentation.
    (C) thorough knowledge of the event.
    (D) to protect self and other EMS personnel.

37. Laws that protect a paramedic if he or she acts in good faith, is not negligent, acts within his or her scope of practice, and does not accept payment for service constitutes the
    (A) implied consent laws.
    (B) Good Samaritan laws.
    (C) malfeasance laws.
    (D) absolute immunity laws.

38. Commonly mandated injuries that are reportable to local authorities include all of the following except
    (A) falls greater than 10 feet.
    (B) child abuse or neglect.
    (C) animal bites.
    (D) gunshot/stab wounds.

39. You and your partner are overheard in the elevator discussing a patient's injuries from a motor vehicle crash. Your conversation included pertinent personal and medical information about the patient. A call was placed to your supervisor because
    (A) you failed to keep patient confidentiality.
    (B) you failed to discuss the appropriate medical care.
    (C) you failed to speak loud enough.
    (D) you failed to recall the injuries correctly.

40. Intentional false communication that injures another person's reputation or good name is a definition of
    (A) invasion of privacy.
    (B) breach of confidentiality.
    (C) informed slander.
    (D) defamation.

41. Personal protective equipment used to operate safely in the rescue environment includes all of the following except
    (A) head protection.
    (B) eye protection.
    (C) hand protection.
    (D) throat and neck protection.

42. It is generally considered unsafe to walk in fast-moving water
    _____ deep.
    (A) ankle
    (B) knee
    (C) waist
    (D) chest

43. _____ (is) are considered "drowning machines" due
    to recirculating currents created by water moving over a uniform
    obstruction.
    (A) Low-head dams
    (B) Current-generated dams
    (C) Rapid-moving water
    (D) White water

44. The body responds to cold water by rapidly losing heat. Protective measures
    exist within the body, which stimulates a parasympathetic response, decreas-
    ing heart rate, causing peripheral vasoconstriction, and shunting blood to
    the core. This cold protective response is known as the
    (A) mammalian dive reflex.
    (B) core shunt mechanism.
    (C) cold survival mechanism.
    (D) physiologic shunt response.

45. Of the following, which is not considered an oxygen-deficient environment
    or confined space?
    (A) Basement
    (B) Storage tanks
    (C) Silos
    (D) Underground vaults

46. You are the first unit on the scene of a multiple-vehicle crash. Upon arrival,
    each of the following actions would be appropriate except
    (A) to establish scene command.
    (B) to treat and transport the most critically ill patient.
    (C) the scene sizeup.
    (D) control scene hazards.

47. Which of the following definitions best describes a disaster?
    (A) Motor vehicle collision with two to three patients
    (B) An everyday incident that generates three or more patients
    (C) A bus or train collision with 25–30 injured
    (D) An incident that overwhelms resources and may damage the infrastruc-
        ture of a region

48. You are assigned the duties of safety officer under the incident command of a local mass casualty incident. You understand the responsibilities of this position to
    (A) monitor all on-scene actions to ensure no potentially harmful situations are created.
    (B) coordinate all operations of this incident that involve outside agencies.
    (C) collect data regarding the incident and relay information to the press or media.
    (D) act as an officer who supervises a specific safety unit or area.

49. The "S" in the acronym START stands for
    (A) suitable.
    (B) simple.
    (C) salvageable.
    (D) sorting.

50. You are the triage officer at a car versus bus collision. Your first victim is approximately 30 years old, awake, alert, and oriented. He is the driver of the car that collided with the bus head on. He complains of lower abdominal pain and has obvious deformity to both femurs. Respirations 24, pulse 140, BP 80/palpated, capillary refill >2 sec. How would you triage the following patient?
    (A) Green
    (B) Yellow
    (C) Red
    (D) Black

51. You are assessing a patient involved in a two-car MVC with severe blunt trauma to the abdomen. You suspect internal hemorrhage. The patient's BP is 100/52 with a pulse rate of 130. You know the elevation in the heart rate is the body's attempt to maintain
    (A) metabolism.
    (B) system integration.
    (C) homeostasis.
    (D) end-organ damage.

52. The movement of water across a cell membrane is known as
    (A) oncotic pressure.
    (B) osmosis.
    (C) diffusion.
    (D) osmolarity.

53. You are treating a patient with diabetic ketoacidosis. The patient is tachy-cardic and has deep, rapid respirations. The most likely cause for the deep, rapid respirations is that
    (A) the body is compensating for a low pH by increasing respirations.
    (B) the body is compensating for a high pH by increasing respirations.
    (C) the body is compensating for an excess of HCO_3 by increasing respirations.
    (D) the body is compensating for a decrease in H^+ ions by increasing respirations.

54. You are treating a patient with hyperventilation syndrome due to an anxiety attack. Which acid-base derangement will hyperventilation produce?
    (A) Respiratory acidosis
    (B) Metabolic acidosis
    (C) Respiratory alkalosis
    (D) Metabolic alkalosis

55. _____ are the primary solutions used for intravenous therapy in the prehospital setting.
    (A) Colloids
    (B) Blood products
    (C) Hypotonic solutions
    (D) Crystalloids

56. The Controlled Substance Act of 1970 created five schedules of controlled substances. Schedule 1 drugs are those drugs with
    (A) accepted medical indications, low potential for abuse and dependence.
    (B) accepted medical indications, high potential for abuse or dependence.
    (C) no accepted medical indications, high potential for abuse and dependence.
    (D) accepted medical indications, less abuse potential and low to moderate physical dependence potential.

57. You are administering amiodarone 300 mg to a patient in full cardiac arrest with a rhythm of ventricular fibrillation. As you start to administer the drug through the endotracheal tube, your partner stops you. Which of the six rights of medication administration were you about to violate?
    (A) Right dose
    (B) Right medication
    (C) Right patient
    (D) Right route

58. Parenteral routes of drug administration include all of the following except
    (A) sublingual.
    (B) intravenous.
    (C) intramuscular.
    (D) topical.

59. A 53-year-old female who is being treated for chronic pain with morphine sulfate continues to complain of pain despite taking her medications as prescribed. The patient is most likely experiencing what response to this medication?
    (A) Allergic reaction
    (B) Tolerance
    (C) Dependence
    (D) Antagonism

60. The desired effects of bronchodilation from the administration of albuterol is the result of stimulation of the_____ receptors in the sympathetic nervous system.
    (A) alpha-1
    (B) alpha-2
    (C) beta-1
    (D) beta-2

61. The standards known as _____ are a major influence on safety standards, standardizing the look and manufacturing designs of ambulances.
    (A) medical equipment standards
    (B) essential equipment standards
    (C) DOT KKK 1822 D specs
    (D) gold standard

62. The type of ambulance that is a standard van with forward control integral cab body is a
    (A) Type I ambulance.
    (B) Type II ambulance.
    (C) Type III ambulance.
    (D) medium-duty ambulance.

63. This agency is involved in the protection of safety for workers including ensuring ambulances are disinfected properly, have sharps containers, and red trash bags.
    (A) OSHA
    (B) FCC
    (C) SOP
    (D) NHTSA

64. At the scene of an MVC your ambulance should be parked at least 100 feet from the accident, uphill and upwind to ensure
    (A) the safety of the vehicle.
    (B) the safety of your crew.
    (C) that the crime scene is not violated.
    (D) clear distance for secondary units to arrive.

65. The following statements regarding scene safety with regard to helicopter and air medical transport are all true except:
    (A) Generally a helicopter requires a landing zone of approximately 100 feet by 100 feet.
    (B) Approach a helicopter from the rear, nearest the tail rotor for safe loading and unloading.
    (C) Ensure that the landing zone is clear of wires, loose debris, towers, or vehicles.
    (D) Mark the landing zone with a single flare and do not shine lights directly into the pilot's eyes.

66. Promptly recognizing the need for emergency management, assessing the scene for danger, contacting Dispatch to mobilize other units for care and transportation of the patient, establishing rapport with the patient and other paramedics on the scene represent the paramedic's
    (A) ethical responsibility.
    (B) roles.
    (C) triage criteria.
    (D) care responsibility.

67. In the mnemonic C-FLOP, when describing the practices of the Incident Management System, the "O" stands for
    (A) operations.
    (B) ongoing assessment.
    (C) order of command.
    (D) officer in charge.

Questions 68–70 are based on the following scenario:
You are assigned to triage patients at the scene of an explosion in a park. You are using the METTAG system of triage.

68. The first victim you come in contact with has no palpable pulse and no respiratory effort. The patient has a major laceration of the scalp with an open skull fracture. You would tag this person as
(A) Green.
(B) Yellow.
(C) Red.
(D) Black.

69. The next patient with whom you come into contact is a 34-year-old female who is wandering around the incident looking for her three-year-old daughter. The patient has multiple abrasions to her face and arms. You would most likely triage this patient
(A) Green.
(B) Yellow.
(C) Red.
(D) Black.

70. The third patient you find is awake, alert, and oriented. The patient has tachypnea with shallow respirations. Your assessment reveals a sucking chest wound on the right side of the chest, a fracture of the right femur, and a large laceration on the forehead. You will most likely triage this patient
(A) Green.
(B) Yellow.
(C) Red.
(D) Black.

71. You and your partner are the first EMS units to arrive on the scene of a single-car MVC, car versus pole. Electrical lines are down across the car. One victim is trapped inside the vehicle. Which action would be most correct?
(A) Immobilize the patient's cervical spine and do a rapid extrication ensuring that the patient does not touch the downed wires.
(B) Control the airway and cervical spine manually while awaiting other units to arrive for proper extrication.
(C) Contact Dispatch and have the power company turn the power off to the lines prior to attempting rescue of this patient.
(D) Ask the patient to slide himself out of the vehicle through a window, being careful not to touch anything metal while exiting.

72. You are the paramedic in charge of a single patient entrapped in a vehicle that was involved in a head-on crash. The extrication of this patient will require a lengthy period of time. Your responsibility during the time of disentanglement will be that
    (A) no treatment is necessary during extrication.
    (B) management of this patient will remain the same as for other emergency patients. Initiation of assessment and care should be started as soon as possible.
    (C) you should initiate only treatment that will assist in the disentanglement.
    (D) treatment should be limited only to identification of injuries.

73. You are transporting a patient who has been exposed to a hazardous material. You have come into contact with this patient with level D hazmat protection equipment on. You have most likely experienced
    (A) a secondary exposure.
    (B) a primary contamination.
    (C) a tertiary contamination.
    (D) no contamination; this level of hazmat protection is sufficient.

74. The paramedic faces many stress-inducing situations. All of the following are phases of the stress response except
    (A) alarm reaction.
    (B) resistance.
    (C) exhaustion.
    (D) acceptance.

75. While eating lunch at a local eatery, you and your partner are discussing a call you had just completed. The patient's relative who is sitting at the next table overhears your partner talking about the patient's condition. Your partner has violated the patient's
    (A) right to consent.
    (B) right to confidentiality.
    (C) right of refusal of treatment.
    (D) character by defamation.

76. While assessing a patient complaining of abdominal pain, you should first
    _____ then _____ the
    abdomen.
    (A) palpate/auscultate
    (B) inspect/percuss
    (C) inspect/ausculate
    (D) palpate/percuss

77. A 50-year-old male is experiencing an acute exacerbation of asthma. Your partner establishes an IV and you prepare to administer albuterol via a hand-held nebulizer. Your actions are in direct accordance with your local protocol. This type of standing order is considered
    (A) on-line medical direction.
    (B) off-line medical direction.
    (C) closed-control medical direction.
    (D) proactive medical command.

78. You and your partner respond to the home of an elderly gentleman who is unresponsive. Your assessment reveals no respiratory effort, skin that is cool and mottled with obvious pooling, and no palpable pulse. The patient's wife presents a valid Do Not Resuscitate order. All of the actions below would be correct except to
    (A) address the wife using gentle eye contact and choosing appropriate words.
    (B) begin to resuscitate this patient without delay.
    (C) explain to the wife that her loved one has died; do not use terms that can be misinterpreted.
    (D) offer assistance to the survivor(s) if necessary.

79. You are one of many local EMS workers who just completed working the scene of a devastating plane crash that left several hundred people dead or injured. You and your crew are called in for CISD (Critical Incident Stress Debriefing). You understand this to be
    (A) a technique for reducing stress on scene that includes fluid replacement, food services, and change of assignments.
    (B) a formal, structured, planned intervention done by a trained team within 24–72 hours of a posttraumatic event. The team includes mental health workers and peers.
    (C) a spontaneous post-call discussion of the events.
    (D) a short informal meeting that gives the crew a chance to vent and verbalize their feelings about this incident.

80. Your crew is dispatched to the home of an obese woman who has fallen. The general rules for lifting and moving this patient include all of the following except to
    (A) anticipate a lengthy time for backup units to arrive; so move this patient to the best of your ability.
    (B) position the load as close to your body as possible.
    (C) bend your knees; let the large muscles of the legs do the work of lifting.
    (D) take your time; do not hurry, and maintain a wide base of support.

ANSWERS AND ANSWER EXPLANATIONS

1. **(C)** The patient care report may be the only accurate account available to healthcare professionals, as well as other people interested in the event.

2. **(A)** All incident times are to be recorded accurately for legal purposes including time of call, time of dispatch, time of arrival, time of medication administration, etc.

3. **(D)** Pertinent negatives are findings that require no medical treatment but help to show the completeness of the paramedic's history and exam on the PCR.

4. **(B)** To correct an error on a PCR, a single line should be struck through the error with the EMT-Paramedic's initials next to the error and dated.

5. **(B)** The accuracy and completeness of the patient care report may have a significant impact on ongoing care and treatment of the patient.

6. **(A)** The patient's insurance information is not a necessary part of documentation included in a patient care refusal.

7. **(C)** Revisions are acceptable and must be done on a separate form and then attached to the original document.

8. **(A)** Medical terminology is an integral part of good documentation on a PCR.

9. **(B)** A duplex communication system allows the user to both listen and speak at the same time. A simplex system **(A)** allows a person to listen or speak at one time. A multiplex system **(C)** allows a person to listen and speak, as well as transmit data. A trunked system **(D)** pools all frequencies and routes transmissions to the next available frequency.

10. **(D)** Feedback is a vital part of communication, allowing the sender to know that the receiver understands the message.

11. **(A)** Proper terminology helps to make communication clear, concise, and unambiguous.

12. **(A)** In a simplex system the user is able only to listen or speak. The major disadvantages include the fact that the process is slower, more formal, and not facilitating discussion.

13. **(D)** An advantage of cellular telephones include promoting a less formal, shorter discussion of EMS events. Disadvantages include lost or broken signals due to geographical area or cell sites.

14. **(C)** FCC stands for the Federal Communications Commission, which regulates telecommunications in the United States. Functions include licensing, frequency allocation, technical standards, and rule making/enforcement.

15. **(B)** It is not the role of the EMS dispatcher to diagnose the nature of the illness. EMS dispatchers serve by receiving the call, taking information regarding the nature of the event, and providing prearrival instructions to assist prior to the EMS unit's arrival.

16. **(C)** Prearrival instructions provide immediate instructions and assistance to patients prior to arrival of EMS units.

17. **(D)** Bacteria, viruses, and fungi are all examples of infectious agents, which have the potential of causing an infection.

18. **(A)** The skin is the body's first line of defense against infectious agents.

19. **(C)** Making this patient a load and go patient based on the information provided is an inappropriate action.

20. **(A)** Isolation of the HIV patient is an inappropriate action. Care includes being supportive, using appropriate BSI based on the task being performed, effective handwashing, disinfection of equipment, and care in use of equipment, especially sharps.

21. **(A)** Hepatitis A is transmitted via the oral/fecal route.

22. **(C)** Tuberculosis presents with a chronic cough persistent for two to three weeks, low-grade fever, and night sweats. Certain populations are at a higher risk of developing TB including children less than 3 years old and geriatric patients.

23. **(B)** Tuberculosis is transmitted through exposure to airborne droplets, and prolonged close exposure to a person with active TB.

24. **(D)** Meningitis signs and symptoms include a severe headache, vomiting, fever, and chills of sudden onset. The patient may have a petechial rash and usually has muscle rigidity.

25. **(C)** Chicken pox/varicella zoster virus is a member of the herpesvirus group. The herpesvirus group also contains a virus responsible for genital herpes and the common cold sore.

26. **(A)** Exposure includes contact of infectious material with eyes, mouth, exposed mucous membranes, or nonintact skin.

27. **(D)** The Medical Practice Act is legislation that governs the practice of medicine to include rules governing the physician's ability to delegate authority to perform medical acts by the paramedic. This legislation varies from one state to another.

28. **(B)** Standard of care can be established by court testimony, reference to published codes, standard criteria, and standards appropriate for the situation.

29. **(C)** Code of conduct. The four elements of a negligence claim include the duty to act, breach of duty, actual damages, and proximate cause.

30. **(B)** Consent is assumed (implied) from any patient requiring emergency intervention who is physically, mentally, or emotionally unable to provide expressed consent.

31. **(B)** Care for this patient would not require parental consent because the patient is married and therefore an emancipated minor.

32. **(D)** This patient can be treated and transported against his will under involuntary consent. Law enforcement personnel can direct transport and treatment of a patient who is a threat to himself or others.

33. **(D)** Abandonment is the termination of the paramedic-patient relationship without ensuring appropriate care for the patient.

34. **(B)** Battery is the unlawful touching of someone without his or her consent.

35. **(B)** Durable power of attorney for health care or health care proxy, once signed and witnessed, are effective until the patient revokes them.

36. **(D)** The primary responsibility of the paramedic at all scenes is the protection of himself or herself and other EMS personnel.

37. **(B)** Good Samaritan laws protect a paramedic if he or she acts in good faith and is not negligent, acts within his or her scope of practice, and does not accept payment for service.

38. **(A)** Falls of greater than 10 feet are not reportable injuries. Injuries reportable to local authorities include spousal abuse, child abuse or neglect, elder abuse, sexual assault, gunshot/stab wounds, animal bites, and communicable diseases.

39. **(A)** Breach of confidentiality. Any medical or personal information about a patient should not be discussed in public or released without the patient's consent.

40. **(D)** Defamation is intentional false communication that injures another person's reputation or good name. Defamation includes slander, which is verbal, and libel, which is written.

41. **(D)** No specific equipment is designed for throat and neck protection. PPE used to safely operate in rescue operations includes eye protection, head protection, hand protection, personal flotation devices, thermal protection, high visibility clothing, and specialized footwear.

42. **(B)** Knee deep. Walking in fast-moving water places the person at risk of having an extremity pinned and then being pulled under by the current.

43. **(A)** Low-head dams create a recirculating current, which can repeatedly pull the victim under the water, making escape difficult. These dams also make rescue operations hazardous.

44. **(A)** The mammalian dive reflex is a protective physiologic response, which increases survivability by shunting blood to the core, decreasing heart rate, and dropping blood pressure. These factors are affected by the person's age and health status and the water temperature.

45. **(A)** A basement is not an oxygen-deficient environment. Oxygen-deficient/ confined spaces include storage tanks, grain bins or silos, wells, manholes, and underground vaults.

46. **(B)** The first unit to arrive on the scene should begin the scene sizeup, which includes establishing command, calling for back-up units, controlling any hazards, and locating any triage patients. It would not be appropriate for the primary unit to locate and transport the most critically injured patient.

47. **(D)** A disaster is an incident that may generate hundreds of patients, may overwhelm the existing resources, and may damage the infrastructure of the region shutting down railroads, hospitals, and other normal operations.

48. **(A)** The safety officer monitors all on-scene actions to ensure that no potentially harmful situations are created.

49. **(B)** "Simple." START stands for simple triage and rapid transport. This system focuses on four easily identifiable findings: (1) ability to walk, (2) respiratory effort, (3) pulses/perfusion, (4) neurological status.

50. **(C)** This patient should be tagged Red with immediate life threats including the possibility of bilateral femur fractures and intraabdominal bleeding.

51. **(C)** Homeostasis is the natural tendency of the body to maintain a steady state of equilibrium within the body's internal environment.

52. **(B)** Osmosis is the movement of any solvent (usually water) across a cell membrane.

53. **(A)** The brain recognizes a decrease in pH or excess of H^+ ions and attempts to compensate by increasing the respiratory effort.

54. **(C)** Respiratory alkalosis results from an increase in respirations and an excessive elimination of CO_2.

55. **(D)** Crystalloids are the primary solutions used for intravenous fluid therapies in the prehospital setting.

56. **(C)** Schedule 1 drugs include heroin, LSD, and mescaline. Schedule 1 drugs pose a high abuse potential and may lead to severe dependence.

57. **(D)** Right route. Amiodarone cannot be given via the endotracheal route. The six rights of medication administration include right medication, right dose, right time, right route, right patient, and right documentation.

58. **(A)** Parenteral routes for delivery of medication include all those areas outside the gastrointestinal tract. Parenteral routes include intravenous, endotracheal, intramuscular, subcutaneous, topical, and inhalation. The sublingual route administers the drug through the enteral route, or through the gastrointestinal tract.

59. **(B)** Tolerance is a decreased response to the same amount of a drug after taking the drug over a period of time.

60. **(D)** The stimulation of beta-2 receptors causes bronchodilation, dilatation of arterioles, inhibition of uterine contractions, and skeletal muscle tremors.

61. **(C)** The DOT KKK 1822 D specs outline the design and manufacturing specifications produced by the Federal General Services Administrative Automotive Commodity Center.

62. **(B)** Type II is a standard van-type ambulance. The Type I ambulance is the design of a conventional truck cab chassis with a modular ambulance body. Type III is a specialty van with the larger cab body ambulance. The medium-duty ambulance is a larger vehicle designed to handle heavier loads.

63. **(A)** OSHA stands for Occupational Safety and Health Administration. This agency is charged with protecting worker safety.

64. **(B)** The number one priority of every EMS call is assurance of your personal safety.

65. **(B)** The helicopter should cautiously be approached in a crouched position away from the tail rotor. Approach a helicopter that is on a slight incline from the downhill side.

66. **(B)** Roles: Recognizing an emergency exists, assessing the situation, managing the emergency care, coordinating efforts of your team as well as other agencies involved in the care and transportation of the patient, and establishing rapport with the patient and other EMS crew are all examples of a paramedic's roles.

67. **(A)** The mnemonic C-FLOP stands for: C—command; F—finance/administration; L—logistics; O—operations; P—planning.

68. **(D)** Black. The designation of this patient would be black due to the absence of signs of life and injuries that were possibly incompatible with life. The morgue area should be a triage area away from other treatment areas.

69. **(A)** Green. This patient can be triaged to the green treatment area. The green treatment area is the area where patients require little or no care in preparation for transport.

70. **(C)** Red. This patient has critical injuries that require immediate attention. The red treatment area has the equipment and skilled providers to best care for, stabilize, and transport this patient.

71. **(C)** The rescuer's top priority is the safety of himself or herself and other rescuers. Attempting any rescue prior to cutting power to the downed lines would jeopardize the safety of the rescuers and the patient.

72. **(B)** Keep in mind that rapid extrication and transport may not be possible. Management of this patient should remain the same as similar emergency patients. You must initiate assessment and care as soon as possible.

73. **(A)** For a secondary contamination level D hazmat protection equipment is the lowest level of protection. Level D equipment consists of structural firefighting, or turn-out gear. Secondary contamination **(A)** occurs when an uncontaminated person comes in contact with a contaminated person.

74. **(D)** The three phases of the body's response to stress are alarm reaction (or the fight or flight response) **(A)**; resistance **(B)** and as the body sustains increasing stress the level of resistance to stress rises and higher levels of stress must occur for the alarm reaction to occur; exhaustion **(C)** as stress continues coping mechanisms begin to fail.

75. **(B)** Information related to the patient's condition or treatment is considered confidential information.

76. **(C)** Inspection is the visual assessment of the patient. Inspection can reveal many important aspects of the patient. Auscultation of abdominal sounds should precede palpation and percussion.

77. **(B)** Off-line medical direction includes the authority of a medical director or advisory group to establish treatment protocols or standing orders.

78. **(B)** This patient has a valid DNR (Do Not Resuscitate) order and no obvious signs of life. The correct actions would be to address the survivor in terms that leave no doubt about the outcome of the deceased. Use gentle reassuring eye contact and offer any assistance that may be needed to the survivor.

79. **(B)** CISD is a formal, structured, planned intervention performed by a CISM (critical incident stress management) team, which includes mental health workers and peers. The intervention should take place within 24–72 hours after a posttraumatic event.

80. **(A)** Proper lifting techniques should be utilized during all patient encounters. Ask for assistance if needed; do not jeopardize the rescuer or patient's safety.

Notes

Notes

Practice Test 1

As mentioned in Chapter One, most students will complete the National Registry exam in 70–100 questions, but in some cases students may answer up to 120 questions.

This practice exam contains 120 questions. This will help prepare you in case you end up taking a long exam. This exam is not divided into individual sections or chapters. The questions are in random order to mirror the layout of the National Registry Exam.

You should allow yourself 120 minutes (1 minute per question). This will give you a realistic idea of how you will need to pace yourself.

Hold yourself to a high standard for this practice exam by scoring 85% or better. This is achievable by answering 96 questions correctly.

All ECG strips used in this practice exam are six-second strips.

When you complete this exam, move on to the CD that contains two additional practice exams.

Answer Sheet
PRACTICE TEST 1

1 Ⓐ Ⓑ Ⓒ Ⓓ	31 Ⓐ Ⓑ Ⓒ Ⓓ	61 Ⓐ Ⓑ Ⓒ Ⓓ	91 Ⓐ Ⓑ Ⓒ Ⓓ
2 Ⓐ Ⓑ Ⓒ Ⓓ	32 Ⓐ Ⓑ Ⓒ Ⓓ	62 Ⓐ Ⓑ Ⓒ Ⓓ	92 Ⓐ Ⓑ Ⓒ Ⓓ
3 Ⓐ Ⓑ Ⓒ Ⓓ	33 Ⓐ Ⓑ Ⓒ Ⓓ	63 Ⓐ Ⓑ Ⓒ Ⓓ	93 Ⓐ Ⓑ Ⓒ Ⓓ
4 Ⓐ Ⓑ Ⓒ Ⓓ	34 Ⓐ Ⓑ Ⓒ Ⓓ	64 Ⓐ Ⓑ Ⓒ Ⓓ	94 Ⓐ Ⓑ Ⓒ Ⓓ
5 Ⓐ Ⓑ Ⓒ Ⓓ	35 Ⓐ Ⓑ Ⓒ Ⓓ	65 Ⓐ Ⓑ Ⓒ Ⓓ	95 Ⓐ Ⓑ Ⓒ Ⓓ
6 Ⓐ Ⓑ Ⓒ Ⓓ	36 Ⓐ Ⓑ Ⓒ Ⓓ	66 Ⓐ Ⓑ Ⓒ Ⓓ	96 Ⓐ Ⓑ Ⓒ Ⓓ
7 Ⓐ Ⓑ Ⓒ Ⓓ	37 Ⓐ Ⓑ Ⓒ Ⓓ	67 Ⓐ Ⓑ Ⓒ Ⓓ	97 Ⓐ Ⓑ Ⓒ Ⓓ
8 Ⓐ Ⓑ Ⓒ Ⓓ	38 Ⓐ Ⓑ Ⓒ Ⓓ	68 Ⓐ Ⓑ Ⓒ Ⓓ	98 Ⓐ Ⓑ Ⓒ Ⓓ
9 Ⓐ Ⓑ Ⓒ Ⓓ	39 Ⓐ Ⓑ Ⓒ Ⓓ	69 Ⓐ Ⓑ Ⓒ Ⓓ	99 Ⓐ Ⓑ Ⓒ Ⓓ
10 Ⓐ Ⓑ Ⓒ Ⓓ	40 Ⓐ Ⓑ Ⓒ Ⓓ	70 Ⓐ Ⓑ Ⓒ Ⓓ	100 Ⓐ Ⓑ Ⓒ Ⓓ
11 Ⓐ Ⓑ Ⓒ Ⓓ	41 Ⓐ Ⓑ Ⓒ Ⓓ	71 Ⓐ Ⓑ Ⓒ Ⓓ	101 Ⓐ Ⓑ Ⓒ Ⓓ
12 Ⓐ Ⓑ Ⓒ Ⓓ	42 Ⓐ Ⓑ Ⓒ Ⓓ	72 Ⓐ Ⓑ Ⓒ Ⓓ	102 Ⓐ Ⓑ Ⓒ Ⓓ
13 Ⓐ Ⓑ Ⓒ Ⓓ	43 Ⓐ Ⓑ Ⓒ Ⓓ	73 Ⓐ Ⓑ Ⓒ Ⓓ	103 Ⓐ Ⓑ Ⓒ Ⓓ
14 Ⓐ Ⓑ Ⓒ Ⓓ	44 Ⓐ Ⓑ Ⓒ Ⓓ	74 Ⓐ Ⓑ Ⓒ Ⓓ	104 Ⓐ Ⓑ Ⓒ Ⓓ
15 Ⓐ Ⓑ Ⓒ Ⓓ	45 Ⓐ Ⓑ Ⓒ Ⓓ	75 Ⓐ Ⓑ Ⓒ Ⓓ	105 Ⓐ Ⓑ Ⓒ Ⓓ
16 Ⓐ Ⓑ Ⓒ Ⓓ	46 Ⓐ Ⓑ Ⓒ Ⓓ	76 Ⓐ Ⓑ Ⓒ Ⓓ	106 Ⓐ Ⓑ Ⓒ Ⓓ
17 Ⓐ Ⓑ Ⓒ Ⓓ	47 Ⓐ Ⓑ Ⓒ Ⓓ	77 Ⓐ Ⓑ Ⓒ Ⓓ	107 Ⓐ Ⓑ Ⓒ Ⓓ
18 Ⓐ Ⓑ Ⓒ Ⓓ	48 Ⓐ Ⓑ Ⓒ Ⓓ	78 Ⓐ Ⓑ Ⓒ Ⓓ	108 Ⓐ Ⓑ Ⓒ Ⓓ
19 Ⓐ Ⓑ Ⓒ Ⓓ	49 Ⓐ Ⓑ Ⓒ Ⓓ	79 Ⓐ Ⓑ Ⓒ Ⓓ	109 Ⓐ Ⓑ Ⓒ Ⓓ
20 Ⓐ Ⓑ Ⓒ Ⓓ	50 Ⓐ Ⓑ Ⓒ Ⓓ	80 Ⓐ Ⓑ Ⓒ Ⓓ	110 Ⓐ Ⓑ Ⓒ Ⓓ
21 Ⓐ Ⓑ Ⓒ Ⓓ	51 Ⓐ Ⓑ Ⓒ Ⓓ	81 Ⓐ Ⓑ Ⓒ Ⓓ	111 Ⓐ Ⓑ Ⓒ Ⓓ
22 Ⓐ Ⓑ Ⓒ Ⓓ	52 Ⓐ Ⓑ Ⓒ Ⓓ	82 Ⓐ Ⓑ Ⓒ Ⓓ	112 Ⓐ Ⓑ Ⓒ Ⓓ
23 Ⓐ Ⓑ Ⓒ Ⓓ	53 Ⓐ Ⓑ Ⓒ Ⓓ	83 Ⓐ Ⓑ Ⓒ Ⓓ	113 Ⓐ Ⓑ Ⓒ Ⓓ
24 Ⓐ Ⓑ Ⓒ Ⓓ	54 Ⓐ Ⓑ Ⓒ Ⓓ	84 Ⓐ Ⓑ Ⓒ Ⓓ	114 Ⓐ Ⓑ Ⓒ Ⓓ
25 Ⓐ Ⓑ Ⓒ Ⓓ	55 Ⓐ Ⓑ Ⓒ Ⓓ	85 Ⓐ Ⓑ Ⓒ Ⓓ	115 Ⓐ Ⓑ Ⓒ Ⓓ
26 Ⓐ Ⓑ Ⓒ Ⓓ	56 Ⓐ Ⓑ Ⓒ Ⓓ	86 Ⓐ Ⓑ Ⓒ Ⓓ	116 Ⓐ Ⓑ Ⓒ Ⓓ
27 Ⓐ Ⓑ Ⓒ Ⓓ	57 Ⓐ Ⓑ Ⓒ Ⓓ	87 Ⓐ Ⓑ Ⓒ Ⓓ	117 Ⓐ Ⓑ Ⓒ Ⓓ
28 Ⓐ Ⓑ Ⓒ Ⓓ	58 Ⓐ Ⓑ Ⓒ Ⓓ	88 Ⓐ Ⓑ Ⓒ Ⓓ	118 Ⓐ Ⓑ Ⓒ Ⓓ
29 Ⓐ Ⓑ Ⓒ Ⓓ	59 Ⓐ Ⓑ Ⓒ Ⓓ	89 Ⓐ Ⓑ Ⓒ Ⓓ	119 Ⓐ Ⓑ Ⓒ Ⓓ
30 Ⓐ Ⓑ Ⓒ Ⓓ	60 Ⓐ Ⓑ Ⓒ Ⓓ	90 Ⓐ Ⓑ Ⓒ Ⓓ	120 Ⓐ Ⓑ Ⓒ Ⓓ

1. You arrive on the scene of a two-car MVC. The driver of the first vehicle is unconscious. Consent for this patient is said to be
   (A) informed.
   (B) implied.
   (C) expressed.
   (D) involuntary.

2. You are caring for a victim of a motor vehicle collision who has sustained multiple traumatic injuries. You are in a region in which the trauma care system consists of a Level I trauma center 50 minutes away and a Level III trauma center 10 minutes away. What is your choice of treatment facilities and why?
   (A) Level I trauma center because it is the only center that is truly capable of handling trauma cases
   (B) Level I trauma center because you may be held liable if you take the patient to a facility of lesser capability
   (C) Level III trauma center because it is capable of handling all types of specialty trauma
   (D) Level III trauma center because it will stabilize and transfer serious patients as needed as part of a trauma system

3. Laws that protect a paramedic if he or she acts in good faith, is not negligent, acts within his or her scope of practice, and does not accept payment for service are called
   (A) implied consent laws.
   (B) Good Samaritan laws.
   (C) malfeasance laws.
   (D) absolute immunity laws.

4. Vasopressin is indicated for management of
   (A) any circumstance in which epinephrine 1:10,000 may be used.
   (B) ventricular fibrillation.
   (C) PEA.
   (D) ventricular tachycardia with a pulse.

5. What is the first pharmacological agent to be administered in a pediatric cardiac arrest?
   (A) Atropine 1.0 mg
   (B) Epinephrine 1:10,000
   (C) Lidocaine 1 mg/kg
   (D) Epinephrine 1:1,000

6. You have a patient who presents with a whole-body rash. There is no complaint of shortness of breath. Which of the following history findings lead you to conclude that the rash is the result of a delayed hypersensitivity reaction?
   (A) History of eating shellfish 30 minutes ago
   (B) History of taking a new medication for the past seven days
   (C) History of insect sting last summer
   (D) History of chlamydia

7. You have arrived on scene where you find a 50-year-old male who has a large jagged laceration from a chain saw on his medial left upper thigh. Bright red blood is spurting from the wound. Your patient is alert, oriented, and anxious, with pale, diaphoretic skin. What is the priority of care for this patient?
   (A) Two large-bore IVs wide open
   (B) Immobilization of the c-spine and preparation to intubate
   (C) Tourniquet of the upper right leg
   (D) Application of a pressure dressing while elevating the left leg

8. The minimum chest compression rate for a two-year-old in cardiac arrest is
   (A) 80/minute.
   (B) 100/minute.
   (C) 110/minute.
   (D) 120/minute.

9. A bag-valve mask device with a reservoir and an adequate oxygen source (at least 15 LPM) will deliver an oxygen concentration of
   (A) 21%.
   (B) 40% to 60%.
   (C) 80%.
   (D) 100%.

10. A 30-year-old suddenly developed a two- to three-minute grand mal seizure. On scene you find an unconscious and unresponsive patient. After the insertion of an oropharyngeal airway, applying high-flow oxygen, and assisting ventilations with a bag-valve mask, the patient's pulse oximetry reading is 90%. His skin is pale and moist. It is important to consider
    (A) a paralyzed diaphragm.
    (B) transport to a hospital.
    (C) endotracheal intubation.
    (D) placement of a nasopharyngeal airway.

11. It is important to avoid *excessively* hyperventilating a head injury patient because it can
    (A) increase the blood $PaCO_2$ to dangerously high levels.
    (B) decrease the blood $PaCO_2$ to dangerously low levels.
    (C) cause jugular vein distention.
    (D) vasodilate the brain's vasculature.

12. A patient is exhibiting decorticate posturing to painful stimuli. These are signs that indicate
    (A) decreased peripheral perfusion.
    (B) a lesion of the spinal cord.
    (C) decreased $PaCO_2$ blood levels.
    (D) a lesion at or above the upper brain stem.

13. The recommended dose of amiodarone in a pediatric patient with ventricular fibrillation is
    (A) 5 mg.
    (B) 150 mg.
    (C) 0.5 mg/kg.
    (D) 5 mg/kg.

14. A patient is experiencing severe chest pain and dyspnea. He is nauseated and extremely diaphoretic, BP is 78/42, pulse is tachycardic, respirations are 36. The patient weighs 190 pounds. ECG shows the following rhythm:

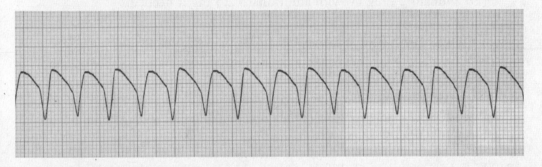

    Initial treatment should include
    (A) lidocaine 85 to 130 mg IVP.
    (B) defibrillation.
    (C) cardioversion.
    (D) Adenocard 6 mg rapid IVP.

15. Hyperventilation resulting from pure anxiety leads to
    (A) respiratory acidosis.
    (B) respiratory alkalosis.
    (C) a decreasing blood pH.
    (D) hepatic failure.

16. Signs and symptoms associated with pericardial tamponade include distant heart tones, JVD, and
    (A) pulse paradoxus.
    (B) hypotension.
    (C) wheezing.
    (D) delayed capillary refill.

17. You are caring for a child with respiratory distress. You note a harsh high-pitched sound with each breath. You suspect this is indicative of
    (A) stridor.
    (B) wheezing.
    (C) crackles.
    (D) rhonchi.

18. Pain with palpation under the right costal margin is known as
    (A) McBurney's point.
    (B) Murphy's sign.
    (C) Grey-Turner's sign.
    (D) Cullen's sign.

19. Pain medication indicated for acute cholecystitis is
    (A) morphine 2–10 mg IV titrated for pain relief.
    (B) Demerol 25–50 mg IV titrated for pain relief.
    (C) fentanyl 25–50 mg IV one time only.
    (D) Nubain 25 mg IV with additional 12.5 mg if needed.

20. Cushing's reflex includes a sudden increase in systolic pressure, bradycardia, and
    (A) erratic respirations.
    (B) irregular pulse.
    (C) increased respirations.
    (D) pupil dilation.

21. Lidocaine may be lethal if administered to a patient with which of the following dysrhythmias?
    (A) Sinus rhythm with PACs
    (B) Second-degree AV block type I
    (C) Accelerated junctional rhythm
    (D) Second-degree AV block type II

22. What is the ratio of chest compressions to ventilations when performing one-person CPR on an adult?
    (A) 5 compressions to 1 ventilation
    (B) 15 compressions to 2 ventilations
    (C) 30 compressions to 2 ventilations
    (D) 5 compressions to 2 ventilations

23. Field extubation is indicated if the patient
    (A) is awake and able to maintain his or her own airway.
    (B) is unconscious and continually bites the endotracheal tube.
    (C) is not suspected of alcohol intoxication.
    (D) becomes combative and starts to delay additional treatment.

24. You have just delivered a full-term baby in the back of your ambulance. The initial APGAR score is 5. Treatment should consist of
(A) CPR.
(B) effective ventilation.
(C) vascular access.
(D) administration of epinephrine.

25. The paramedic faces many stress-inducing situations. All of the following are phases of the stress response EXCEPT
(A) alarm reaction.
(B) resistance.
(C) exhaustion.
(D) acceptance.

26. Your EMS team is dispatched to care for a 39-year-old female with difficulty breathing. She is awake and appears restless and apprehensive. Her vital signs are: BP 148/92; radial pulse strong at 124; respirations 36 and shallow. Her skin is pale, cool, and dry. She denies having chest pain or any health problems. Your patient's pulse oximetry reading is 89% on room air. This indicates that
(A) she is breathing too deeply.
(B) she is breathing within normal limits.
(C) she has hypoxemia.
(D) she has psychogenically induced hyperventilation syndrome.

27. During your interview of a patient with dyspnea, you find that the patient takes birth control pills and has had left calf tenderness for two days with no history of trauma to the area. This information leads you to suspect
(A) viral pneumonia.
(B) pulmonary edema.
(C) a panic attack.
(D) a pulmonary embolus.

28. You interpret this cardiac rhythm as

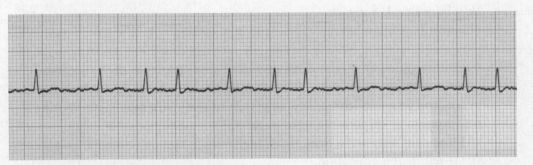

(A) junctional tachycardia.
(B) sinus tachycardia with premature atrial contractions (PACs).
(C) atrial fibrillation with a rapid ventricular response.
(D) superventricular tachycardia.

29. What is the correct speed at which you should perform chest compressions on an adult victim of cardiac arrest?
    (A) 100 times per minute
    (B) 60 times per minute
    (C) 120 times per minute
    (D) 80 times per minute

30. You respond to a "man down" call. When you arrive, you find a 52-year-old male patient lying on the ground next to a ladder. It is unclear if he was placing the ladder against the house when it came into contact with power lines or if he fell from the top of the ladder. Examination shows the patient to be unresponsive. He has a rapid irregular pulse and snoring respirations at 8; BP is 88/42. Treatment should include
    (A) assisted ventilation with a bag-valve device at 6–10 LPM.
    (B) assisted ventilation with a nonrebreather mask at 10–15 LPM.
    (C) opening the airway with a jaw-thrust maneuver and ventilation with a bag-valve device.
    (D) insertion of an oropharyngeal airway and oxygen by nonrebreather mask at 10–15 LPM.

31. A patient has a complaint of chest pain. BP is 160/90, pulse 46, and respirations 20. You apply a cardiac monitor and note the following rhythm:

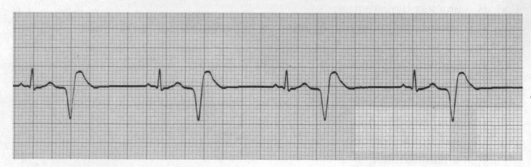

    Treatment includes
    (A) atropine 0.5 mg.
    (B) immediate defibrillation.
    (C) lidocaine 1.5 mg/kg.
    (D) continued observation.

32. Communication from the EMS dispatcher that provides the caller with emotional support, may be life sustaining to the patient during a critical event, and provides immediate assistance to the caller as well as ongoing information to responding units is called
    (A) incident data collection.
    (B) predispatch education.
    (C) prearrival instructions.
    (D) incident referral data.

33. Physical assessment findings, signs, or symptoms that support your suspicion that a patient is under the influence of alcohol *or* drugs include

1. chest pain and dysrhythmias
2. confusion and polyuria
3. dilated pupils and anxiety
4. constricted pupils and respiratory depression

(A) 1 and 2
(B) 2 and 3
(C) 2, 3, and 4
(D) All of the above

34. After defibrillating a patient with pulseless ventricular tachycardia, the first medication you should give is
(A) epinephrine or vasopressin.
(B) lidocaine or amiodarone.
(C) epinephrine or lidocaine.
(D) vasopressin or amiodarone.

35. In a pediatric patient, initial cardioversion should be performed at
(A) 0.5–1.0 J/kg.
(B) 4 J/kg.
(C) 2 J/kg.
(D) 100 J.

36. Manual maneuvers used to open a patient's airway
(A) are contraindicated in most patients.
(B) are difficult to perform.
(C) include head-tilt/chin-lift and jaw thrust.
(D) do not usually work without more extensive intervention.

37. Your patient was struck in the head with a six-inch-diameter tree branch while trimming a tree. He complained of dizziness immediately after the incident but states he "feels fine" now. The next day, he complains of dizziness and vomiting. You suspect
(A) an epidural hematoma.
(B) a subdural hematoma.
(C) a concussion.
(D) a contusion.

38. Management of chest pain of a suspected cardiac nature includes
(A) establishing an IV and providing a 200 cc fluid bolus.
(B) administering Lasix 100 mg slow IV.
(C) administering 2 liters oxygen by nasal cannula.
(D) administering nitroglycerin gr1/150 sublingual.

39. The paramedic's primary responsibility at a crime scene or accident scene is
    (A) quality patient care.
    (B) quality documentation.
    (C) thorough knowledge of the event.
    (D) to protect self and other EMS personnel.

40. Supine hypotension syndrome occurs from
    (A) reduction of cardiac output due to compression of the aorta.
    (B) reduction of cardiac output due to compression of the inferior vena cava.
    (C) reduction of cardiac output due to compression of the superior vena cava.
    (D) the uterus pushing up on the diaphragm.

41. A properly written patient care report is important because
    (A) the PCR relays the paramedic's true opinion of the patient.
    (B) the PCR provides the receiving hospital with important billing information.
    (C) the PCR may be the only source for pertinent information for receiving healthcare professionals.
    (D) the PCR links traits of the paramedic with documentation abilities.

42. The simplest airway management technique in a patient *without* suspected cervical spine injury is
    (A) the head-tilt/chin-lift maneuver.
    (B) the modified jaw-thrust maneuver.
    (C) endotracheal intubation.
    (D) nasotracheal intubation.

43. A dissecting aortic aneurysm may produce which of the following signs/symptoms?
    (A) A ripping or tearing pain sensation
    (B) Pain in the abdomen
    (C) The same blood pressure in each arm
    (D) Respiratory distress

44. Revisions to the original patient care report
    (A) should be added on the original document.
    (B) are never appropriate.
    (C) are done on a separate report form and then attached to the original.
    (D) can easily be done in a different color ink.

45. You arrive on scene of a 56-year-old male patient who developed chest pain while mowing the lawn on a hot August day. He states that the pain has subsided after a few minutes of rest. Your assessment shows that he is alert and oriented, BP 148/92, pulse 48, respirations 20. His skin is warm and moist. He has no past medical history and takes no medications. You attach the monitor and observe the following rhythm:

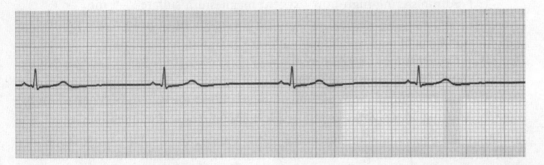

Treatment should include
(A) atropine 0.5 mg IVP.
(B) Adenocard 5 mg IVP.
(C) transport for evaluation.
(D) No treatment is necessary.

46. Your patient suddenly becomes lethargic. His BP is 82/40, pulse 36, respirations 10. You note the following rhythm on the monitor:

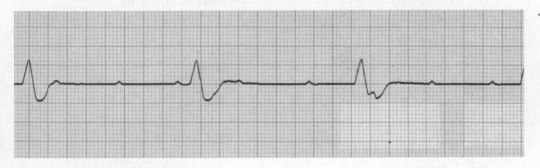

Treatment should include
(A) atropine 0.5 mg IV.
(B) Adenocard 5 mg IV.
(C) stopping nitroglycerin administration.
(D) immediate transcutaneous pacing.

47. You are called to a 32-year-old female who is in her twenty-eighth week of pregnancy. She complains of dizziness, blurred vision, and a feeling that she is going to pass out. Her hands and ankles are edematous and her face is puffy. Vitals are BP 178/108, pulse 104, respirations 24. You are enroute to the hospital when the patient has a grand mal seizure. Treatment for this patient includes
    (A) administering high-flow oxygen, magnesium sulfate 2–5 mg.
    (B) administering oxygen, administering magnesium sulfate 2–5 grams, placing in a right lateral recumbent position.
    (C) maintaining airway, administering oxygen, administering magnesium sulfate 2–5 grams, monitoring vital signs.
    (D) maintaining airway, administering magnesium sulfate 6–8 grams, monitoring vital signs, placing in a left lateral recumbent position.

48. After decompressing the chest of a victim with a tension pneumorthorax, you determine your intervention was successful by observing for
    (A) air rushing from the catheter.
    (B) a decrease in the patient's cyanosis.
    (C) an improvement in the patient's level of consciousness.
    (D) an improvement in the patient's ventilatory and circulatory status.

49. Which of the following statements is true regarding chemical burns?
    (A) Always use antidotes or neutralizing agents.
    (B) Acid burns are typically more serious than alkali burns.
    (C) Both acids and alkalis cause burns by disrupting cell membranes and damaging tissues on contact.
    (D) Always approach a chemical spill from downwind.

50. Procainamide administration should be discontinued if any of the following occur EXCEPT
    (A) hypotension.
    (B) widening of the QRS complex.
    (C) hypertension.
    (D) maximum dose infused.

51. You are called to the scene of a 22-year-old man who was playing in a softball game. He was hit in the eye with a hard-hit line-drive softball. According to his teammates he was knocked to the ground and had a brief loss of consciousness that lasted approximately seven seconds. While assessing the injured eye, you notice a collection of blood in front of the patient's pupil and iris. What is your differential diagnosis?
    (A) Raccoon's eye
    (B) Retinal detachment
    (C) Hyphema
    (D) Corneal laceration

52. You are administering amiodarone 300 mg to a patient in cardiac arrest with a rhythm of ventricular fibrillation. As you start to administer the drug through the endotracheal tube, your partner stops you. Which of the six rights of medication administration were you about to violate?
    (A) Right dose
    (B) Right medication
    (C) Right patient
    (D) Right route

53. All of the following can affect the accuracy reading of a pulse oximeter EXCEPT
    (A) hypoperfusion.
    (B) anemia.
    (C) carbon monoxide poisoning.
    (D) hyperthermia.

54. Sodium bicarbonate administration may be useful for treating
    (A) beta-blocker overdoses and hypocalcemia.
    (B) preexisting acidosis and hypokalemia.
    (C) tricyclic antidepressant overdoses and hyperkalemia.
    (D) calcium channel blocker overdoses and hyperkalemia.

55. The recommended pediatric dose of naloxone for infants and children from birth to five years is
    (A) 20 mg.
    (B) 2.0 mg.
    (C) 0.01 mg/kg.
    (D) 0.1 mg/kg.

56. Applying gentle countertraction to the infant's head to prevent explosive delivery is essential because
    (A) fetal hypoxia can result from rapid delivery.
    (B) if a nuchal cord is present, rapid delivery will make it worse.
    (C) this will allow the perineum to stretch and reduce the chance of tearing.
    (D) the placenta will detach too soon in rapid delivery.

57. The medication treatment of choice for a narrow complex tachycardia in an unstable patient is
    (A) Adenocard.
    (B) lidocaine.
    (C) cardioversion.
    (D) Versed.

58. You are performing rescue breathing with a bag-mask device for an apneic child. How often should you provide rescue breaths?
    (A) Once every 3 seconds
    (B) Once every 4 seconds
    (C) Once every 5 seconds
    (D) Once every 6 seconds

59. A 14-year-old female is crying and hysterical after breaking up with her boyfriend. She had a syncopal episode prior to EMS arrival. Vitals are BP 110/68, pulse 130, and respirations 36. You place her on the cardiac monitor and interpret the following rhythm as

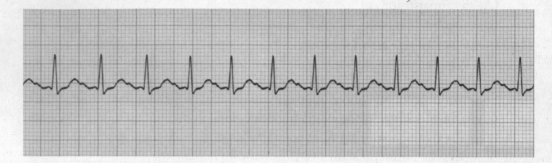

    (A) sinus arrest.
    (B) sinus bradycardia.
    (C) sinus dysrhythmia.
    (D) sinus tachycardia.

60. Choose the best clue for determining possible injuries that may be sustained in an MVC.
    (A) Length of skid marks
    (B) Debris at the scene
    (C) Patient symptoms
    (D) Mechanism of injury

61. You are called to search for an elderly man who wandered from his home. He has been missing for eight hours. It is 38°F outside with a light drizzle. The man is wearing pajamas and slippers. The patient is located lying behind a pile of wood five blocks from his home. He is unconscious, unresponsive, apneic, and pulseless. His skin is cold to the touch and his muscles are rigid. His core body temperature is 89.6°F. Initial treatment should include
    (A) CPR.
    (B) establishing intravenous access with warm normal saline.
    (C) starting passive rewarming.
    (D) pronouncing the patient dead on arrival.

62. You attach the ECG monitor and observe the following rhythm on a hypothermic patient with a core body temperature of 89°F.

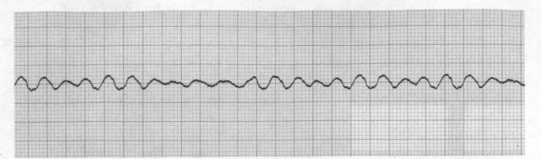

Treatment should include
(A) no treatment until the core temperature is 90°F.
(B) immediate defibrillation.
(C) avoiding rough movement and excessive activity.
(D) Both A and C are correct.

63. You are considering the administration of cardiac medication to a hypothermic patient with a core body temperature of 89°F. Which statement is true?
(A) IV medication may be administered, but spaced at longer than standard intervals.
(B) Withhold medications until the core temperature is 90°F.
(C) IV medications may be administered at regular intervals.
(D) Lidocaine and procainamide will increase the fibrillation threshold.

64. You are sent to evaluate the damage to a vehicle that struck a utility pole head on. Which finding would lead you to believe the patient may have a life-threatening injury?
(A) A deformed dashboard
(B) A deformed steering wheel
(C) An airbag that did not deploy
(D) Significant front end damage

65. It is important to remember that when dealing with an intoxicated patient your assessment must be thorough because
(A) alcohol increases pain tolerance.
(B) alcohol decreases the patient's judgment.
(C) alcohol is a CNS stimulant.
(D) alcohol can mask signs and symptoms of injury.

66. _____ (is) are considered "drowning machines" due to recirculating currents created by water moving over a uniform obstruction.
(A) Low-head dams
(B) Current-generated dams
(C) Rapid-moving water
(D) Whitewater

67. You respond to the home of a patient who has had an unknown illness for two days. You approach the call suspecting an infectious or communicable disease. Which action is not appropriate for this patient's care?
    (A) Gloves and protective eye goggles are worn.
    (B) A full history and detailed physical exam are obtained.
    (C) Make the patient a "load and go" due to the potential for paramedic exposure.
    (D) Disposal of supplies, sharps, appropriately on disposition of the patient.

68. You are assessing a 1½-year-old male with breathing trouble. Inspiratory stridor is heard with evident use of all accessory muscles. The trouble breathing is worse at night. No other significant findings are visible. The child is on no medications and has otherwise been well. You suspect
    (A) epiglottitis.
    (B) asthma.
    (C) bronchiolitis.
    (D) croup.

69. You are treating a 22-year-old female complaining of severe abdominal pain and left shoulder pain. Vital signs are BP 88/64, pulse 128 and regular, respirations of 22, skin cool and wet. She states that she has small amount of pink vaginal discharge. This patient is most likely experiencing
    (A) a ruptured ectopic pregnancy.
    (B) endometriosis.
    (C) pelvic inflammatory disease.
    (D) amenorrhea.

70. You are treating a child with a tension pneumothorax. Needle decompression is needed. The correct site for insertion of the needle is
    (A) below the third rib in the midclavicular line.
    (B) below the second rib in the midaxillary line.
    (C) top of the second rib in the midaxillary line.
    (D) top of the third rib in the midclavicular line.

71. Which of the following rhythms requires immediate transcutaneous pacing?
    (A) Junctional tachycardia
    (B) Sinus bradycardia with first-degree heart block
    (C) Supraventricular tachycardia
    (D) Symptomatic third-degree AV block

72. Which of the following may require synchronized cardioversion?
    (A) Pulseless ventricular tachycardia
    (B) Pulseless electrical activity
    (C) Ventricular fibrillation
    (D) PSVT

73. The proper way to correct a written error on the PCR is to
    (A) use White-Out to cover the error.
    (B) draw a single line through the error, initial, and date the area.
    (C) scribble through the error completely and sign your name next to the error.
    (D) use a black marker to eliminate the error from the PCR, initial, and date the area.

74. A patient experiencing a hypertensive crisis should receive which medication?
    (A) Nitroglycerin
    (B) Procardia
    (C) Aspirin
    (D) Oxygen

75. You are caring for a 78-year-old female patient who has a long history of hyperadrenalism (Cushing's syndrome). She is complaining of left side weakness. You are assigned to establish an IV line and obtain a blood sample for blood glucose testing. You should
    (A) take great care with venipuncture in this patient because hyperadrenalism leads to easy bruising and a delay in healing.
    (B) refuse to establish intravenous access because the veins are fragile and the skin is paper thin.
    (C) not bother checking a blood glucose level because Cushing's syndrome is always associated with hyperglycemia.
    (D) None of the above are correct.

76. While eating lunch at a local eatery, you and your partner are discussing a call you have just completed. The patient's relative, who is sitting at the next table, overhears your partner talking about the patient's condition. Your partner has violated the patient's
    (A) right to consent.
    (B) right to confidentiality.
    (C) right of refusal of treatment.
    (D) character by defamation.

77. You arrive on scene of a 34-year-old male who was struck by a car. Bystanders tell you the patient was standing on the sidewalk when his neighbor, who was backing out of the driveway, struck him. The speed of impact is estimated at less than 5 MPH. Your patient is sitting in the yard with an obvious open tibia/fibula fracture of the right leg. As you auscultate his right upper chest, you notice the patient guarding his shoulder. Closer exam reveals a fractured clavicle. Complications associated with a fractured clavicle include injury to the
    (A) carotid artery.
    (B) subclavian vein.
    (C) descending aorta.
    (D) inferior vena cava.

78. While assessing a trauma patient, you are concerned because his level of consciousness is deteriorating and his heart rate has increased 30 beats per minute. Although his abdomen was unremarkable upon examination, you know that an indicator of severe abdominal trauma is the presence of
    (A) absent bowel sounds.
    (B) back pain.
    (C) referred pain to the clavicle.
    (D) unexplained shock.

79. You are dispatched to a private residence for an eight-year-old boy complaining of trouble breathing. On arrival, you find the patient lethargic with blue lips and rapid labored respirations. He is able to answer questions with only one- or two-word sentences. Physical exam reveals a respiratory rate of 50 per minute; diminished breath sounds and crackles are heard over the right lung field with dullness to percussion. He also has a temperature of 104°F. Based on your assessment, this patient may be experiencing
    (A) cardiogenic shock.
    (B) a drug overdose.
    (C) respiratory distress.
    (D) respiratory failure, most probably due to pneumonia.

80. You and your partner respond to the home of an elderly gentleman who is unresponsive. Your assessment reveals no respiratory effort, skin that is cool and mottled with obvious pooling, and no palpable pulse. The patient's wife presents a valid Do Not Resuscitate order. All of the actions would be correct except to
    (A) address the wife using gentle eye contact and choosing appropriate words.
    (B) begin to resuscitate this patient without delay.
    (C) explain to the wife that her loved one has died; do not use terms that can be misinterpreted.
    (D) offer assistance to the survivor(s) if necessary.

81. The nasopharyngeal airway should be measured
    (A) from the corner of the mouth to the earlobe.
    (B) from the tip of the nose to the earlobe.
    (C) from the tip of the nose to the corner of the mouth.
    (D) from the tip of the nose to the chin.

82. During your assessment of a five-year-old child, you discover a heart rate of 200 beats per minute. The rhythm strip reveals narrow QRS complexes corresponding to the patient's pulse rate. The rhythm most probably represents
    (A) ventricular tachycardia.
    (B) rapid atrial fibrillation.
    (C) supraventricular tachycardia.
    (D) sinus tachycardia.

83. During needle decompression, the needle is inserted on the top of the rib for what purpose?
    (A) To ensure that the vein, artery, and nerve bundle under each rib are not damaged
    (B) To ensure proper placement
    (C) To ensure that the catheter enters the pleural space at the correct angle
    (D) To ensure that the site does not become a sucking chest wound

84. You respond to a 76-year-old man with syncope. He is sitting upright in the bathroom when you arrive. He is initially alert and oriented only to person but quickly regains alertness to person, place, and time. He stated that he was having a bowel movement when he blacked out. You suspect the cause of the patient's syncope is
    (A) digitalis toxicity.
    (B) an atrial dysrhythmia.
    (C) a vasovagal episode.
    (D) underlying myocardial ischemia.

85. All of the following are considered anginal equivalents EXCEPT
    (A) diaphoresis, syncope, dizziness.
    (B) dyspnea, palpitations, syncope.
    (C) hypoglycemia, chest pain, dyspnea.
    (D) fatigue, dizziness, palpitations.

86. Intentional false communication that injures another person's reputation or good name is a definition of
    (A) invasion of privacy.
    (B) breach of confidentiality.
    (C) informed slander.
    (D) defamation.

87. A small child has been struck by a car traveling approximately 25 MPH. The child is unresponsive. The airway maneuver of choice for this patient is
    (A) jaw-thrust with c-spine stabilization.
    (B) head-tilt/chin-lift.
    (C) hyperextension with jaw-thrust.
    (D) hyperflexion of the head to the "sniffing" position.

88. You arrive on the scene of a patient who has been stabbed with a knife in the right side of the back. The patient presents with left-sided hemiparalysis and sensory loss. Despite another stab wound to the right abdomen, the patient denies pain. What type of spinal cord injuries do you suspect?
    (A) Compression
    (B) Transection
    (C) Neurogenic shock
    (D) Brown-Sequard's syndrome

89. The Sellick maneuver
    (A) is used to clear a foreign body airway obstruction in an infant or child.
    (B) is used to clear blood or mucus from an endotracheal tube or the nasopharynx.
    (C) may be used to minimize gastric distention and facilitate placement of an endotracheal tube into the glottic opening.
    (D) is the preferred method for opening the airway of an unconscious patient when cervical spine injury is suspected.

90. You have administered an initial dose of amiodarone for a patient in ventricular fibrillation. The repeat dose of this medication should be
    (A) 300 mg.
    (B) 150 mg.
    (C) 0.04 mg/kg.
    (D) 1 to 1.5 mg/kg.

91. A small child has fallen through the ice while skating. After 30 minutes, the child is pulled from the icy water apneic and pulseless. Your first action in the management of this child should be to
    (A) keep the child cool to maintain the mammalian dive reflex.
    (B) defibrillate the child immediately.
    (C) pronounce the child dead at the scene.
    (D) secure the child's airway and control the cervical spine.

92. Nitroglycerin has all of the following properties EXCEPT that it
    (A) prevents vasospasm.
    (B) is a vasodilator.
    (C) decreases afterload.
    (D) decreases preload.

93. Prompt recognition of the need for emergency management, assessing the scene for danger, contacting Dispatch to mobilize other units for care and transportation of the patient, and establishing rapport with the patient and other paramedics on the scene represent the paramedic's _____:
    (A) ethical responsibility
    (B) roles
    (C) triage criteria
    (D) care responsibility

94. You are the first unit on the scene of a multiple-vehicle crash. Upon arrival, each of the following actions would be appropriate EXCEPT to
    (A) establish scene command.
    (B) treat and transport the most critically ill patient.
    (C) perform a scene sizeup.
    (D) control scene hazards.

95. All of the following are signs and symptoms of organophosphate poisoning EXCEPT
    (A) salivation.
    (B) lacrimation.
    (C) urination.
    (D) tachycardia.

96. You have initiated an IO line in a pediatric patient suffering from severe dehydration. What is the most reliable indicator of successful placement of the IO needle?
    (A) Take an X-ray
    (B) The ability to draw arterial blood through the IO
    (C) Aspiration of bone marrow
    (D) No evidence of fractures after insertion

97. You are assigned the duties of safety officer under the incident command of a mass casualty incident. You understand the responsibilities of this position to be to
    (A) monitor all on-scene actions to ensure that no potentially harmful situations are created.
    (B) coordinate all operations of this incident, which involves outside agencies.
    (C) collect data regarding the incident and relay information to the press or media.
    (D) supervise a specific safety unit or area.

98. Where should you place your hands on the chest of an adult victim when you are performing chest compressions?
    (A) On the top of the sternum
    (B) On the lower one third of the sternum
    (C) On the lower half of the sternum, at the nipple line
    (D) Over the very bottom of the sternum

99. Which one of the following statements is not true regarding electrical injuries?
    (A) Until the power is off, nobody should be allowed to approach the electrical burn patient.
    (B) The rescuer must be grounded to prevent electrical shock when treating a victim of a recent lightning strike.
    (C) Patients in cardiac arrest because of electrocution have a high survival rate if prehospital intervention is prompt.
    (D) Consider the use of 1 mEq/kg of sodium bicarbonate to prevent the complications of rhabdomyolyses.

100. While treating a three-year-old child for amitriptyline ingestion, he suddenly begins to have seizure activity. You decide that administration of diazepam is appropriate. The recommended dose range for this age group is
(A) 0.01–0.02 mg/kg.
(B) 0.05–0.1 mg.
(C) 0.1–0.3 mg/kg.
(D) 5–10 mg.

101. You are dispatched to a 77-year-old male patient who has fallen from a ladder. He fell approximately 14 feet and struck his back on the riding lawn mower as he fell. He is awake and very anxious. He is having obvious trouble breathing. His pulse is 104, respirations 34, and blood pressure 122/76. In your assessment, you find crepitus and instability to the left rib cage. Lung sounds are present and equal. Closer assessment reveals paradoxical chest movement. You suspect
(A) a tension pneumothorax.
(B) a massive hemothorax.
(C) a flail chest.
(D) an abdominal aneurysm.

102. Paradoxical movement is best described as chest wall movement that is
(A) inward with both inspiration and expiration.
(B) inward with expiration and outward with inspiration.
(C) inward with inspiration and outward with expiration.
(D) outward with both inspiration and expiration.

103. Your patient is in severe respiratory distress. Assessment reveals absent lung sounds on the left, tracheal deviation to the right, and an SpO_2 reading of 82%. Immediate treatment must include
(A) intubation.
(B) right side chest decompression.
(C) left side chest decompression.
(D) oxygen administration.

104. You respond to a local physician's office. You are instructed to transport Ms. Smith to the emergency department for acute gastroenteritis. The physician asks you to establish an IV line of normal saline and run it at 100 cc/hr and administer Compazine (prochlorperazine). A proper dose of Compazine for this patient would be
(A) 12.5 mg IV.
(B) 2.5 mg IV.
(C) 10 mg IV.
(D) 1.0 mg IV.

105. You respond to an MVC involving a young child. The child is found apneic but still has a palpable pulse. You immediately begin positive pressure ventilation with a bag-valve mask device. You note that the left side of the chest moves, but the right does not. Lung sounds are absent on the right side and the trachea is deviated to the left. Your immediate action is to
    (A) increase the tidal volume with each ventilation.
    (B) perform a needle decompression on the left side.
    (C) give a 20 cc/kg bolus of IV fluids.
    (D) perform a needle decompression on the right side.

106. Select the statement that correctly relates to pediatric seizures.
    (A) Febrile seizures correlate to the speed in which the temperature rises, not to the degree of the fever.
    (B) Always suspect a fever to be the cause of a seizure if the temperature is more than 101°F.
    (C) Infants and children between the ages of four months and eight years commonly suffer from febrile seizures.
    (D) Febrile seizures do not require transport if the patient can be cooled.

107. You have orally intubated a patient. While your partner ventilates the patient with a bag-valve device, you evaluate placement. Auscultation reveals sounds heard over the right chest and an absence of breath sounds over the left chest. Your best course of action would be to
    (A) hyperventilate the patient and prepare the equipment necessary for a surgical cricothyrotomy.
    (B) deflate the endotracheal tube cuff, withdraw the tube 2 cm, reinflate the cuff, and reevaluate breath sounds.
    (C) deflate the endotracheal tube cuff, remove the endotracheal tube, and hyperventilate the patient with a bag-valve device.
    (D) insert a large diameter needle into the fourth or fifth intercostal space, mid-axillary line.

108. Your patient is a 44-year-old female who was burned when a high-temperature water pipe exploded. She has blisters to the chest, abdomen, entire right arm, and front of the right leg. According to the rule of nines, this patient has sustained _____ percent burns.
    (A) 40.5%
    (B) 36%
    (C) 45%
    (D) 31.5%

109. The recommended dose of vasopressin in cardiac arrest due to pulseless VT or VF is
    (A) 20 units IV bolus repeated once in 10 minutes.
    (B) a single IV bolus dose of 40 units.
    (C) 40 units IV bolus repeated once in 10 minutes.
    (D) 300 mg IV.

110. Your patient is 26 years old and 30 weeks pregnant. She is multigravida but nullipara. She complains of sudden severe tearing abdominal pain with some minor vaginal bleeding. Upon careful palpation, her abdomen is very tender and her uterus seems to be tightly contracted. You suspect
    (A) abruptio placenta.
    (B) an ectopic pregnancy.
    (C) a miscarriage.
    (D) placenta previa.

111. Placenta abruption is caused by
    (A) implantation of the fertilized ovum in a fallopian tube.
    (B) the uterus covering the cervical opening.
    (C) premature separation of the placenta from the uterine wall.
    (D) a spontaneous abortion.

112. A multigravida but nullipara pregnancy history includes
    (A) one pregnancy and one birth.
    (B) many pregnancies and one birth.
    (C) one pregnancy and no births.
    (D) many pregnancies and no births.

113. Your EMS team is called to attend to a patient in her mid-thirties who is having a generalized motor seizure. Bystanders inform you that she has been seizing continually for the past 10 minutes. You note that the patient is shaking violently, is diaphoretic, and is slightly cyanotic. An IV is started and the blood glucose reading is 120 mg/dl. A medication and correct dose range that you could administer to her is
    (A) Valium (diazepam) 5–10 mg IVP.
    (B) dextrose 50% in water 5–10 grams.
    (C) Valium (diazepam) 5–10 mcg IVP.
    (D) Versed (midazolam) 10–25 mg IVP.

114. You are called to the scene of a two-year-old child with a three-day history of diarrhea. The child appears to be in no respiratory distress with good breath sounds bilaterally. The heart rate is 140 per minute and the BP is 86/60. Capillary refill is delayed at about 4 seconds. The peripheral pulses are weak. After obtaining vascular access, which of the following would be the next intervention?
    (A) Get a chest X-ray.
    (B) Initiate a dopamine infusion at 2–5 mcg/kg/minute.
    (C) Start oral hydration.
    (D) Administer a 20 cc/kg bolus of normal saline.

115. You are using an end-tidal carbon dioxide detector as a tool to assist for proper endotracheal intubation placement. The absence of carbon dioxide in exhaled air indicates that the endotracheal tube has been
    (A) placed in the right mainstem bronchus.
    (B) correctly placed in the trachea.
    (C) placed in the esophagus.
    (D) placed in the left mainstem bronchus.

116. When using the rule of nines for calculating burns, which of the following is a correct modification for a child?
    (A) The front of each arm for a child is 7% compared to 4½% on an adult.
    (B) The front of each leg for a child is 4½% compared to 9% on an adult.
    (C) The head of a child is 18% compared to 9% on an adult.
    (D) The entire leg of a child is 9% compared to 18% on an adult.

117. Your squad is dispatched to the scene of a six-year-old child with an elevated temperature. The mother tells you that the child was fine last night and got up this morning complaining of a sore throat and trouble swallowing. The initial assessment reveals a sick-looking child who is leaning forward in the tripod position. He is obviously drooling. From this information, you suspect
    (A) bronchiolitis.
    (B) croup.
    (C) epiglottitis.
    (D) meningitis.

118. A 22-year-old female has just finished jogging five miles. She is complaining of palpitations. Vitals are blood pressure, 112/68; pulse, 148; and respirations, 32. She denies drug use. ECG shows the following rhythm:

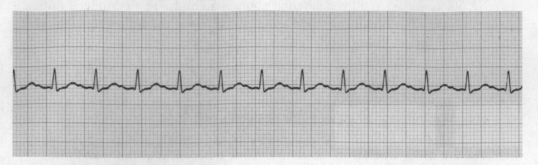

Treatment should include
(A) adenosine 6 mg rapid IVP.
(B) cardioversion at 100 joules.
(C) vagal maneuvers.
(D) continued observation.

119. Hypocalcemia and hypomagnesemia would MOST likely result in
(A) decreased cardiac conduction.
(B) increased myocardial irritability.
(C) decreased cardiac contractility.
(D) decreased myocardial automaticity.

120. When assessing a 12-lead ECG, acute infarction to the inferior wall of the myocardium would present as
(A) pathologic Q waves in leads V_4 and V_5.
(B) ST segment elevation in leads II, III, and aVF.
(C) T-wave inversion in leads V_1 through V_4.
(D) ST segment depression in leads II and III.

Answer Key
PRACTICE TEST 1

1. B	31. D	61. A	91. D
2. D	32. C	62. B	92. C
3. B	33. D	63. A	93. B
4. B	34. A	64. B	94. B
5. B	35. A	65. D	95. D
6. B	36. C	66. A	96. C
7. D	37. B	67. C	97. A
8. B	38. D	68. D	98. C
9. D	39. D	69. A	99. B
10. C	40. B	70. D	100. C
11. B	41. C	71. D	101. C
12. D	42. A	72. D	102. C
13. D	43. A	73. B	103. C
14. C	44. C	74. D	104. C
15. B	45. C	75. A	105. D
16. B	46. D	76. B	106. A
17. A	47. C	77. B	107. B
18. B	48. D	78. D	108. B
19. B	49. C	79. D	109. B
20. A	50. C	80. B	110. A
21. D	51. C	81. B	111. C
22. C	52. D	82. C	112. D
23. A	53. D	83. A	113. A
24. B	54. C	84. C	114. D
25. D	55. D	85. C	115. C
26. C	56. C	86. D	116. C
27. D	57. A	87. A	117. C
28. C	58. D	88. D	118. C
29. A	59. D	89. C	119. B
30. C	60. D	90. B	120. B

ANSWER EXPLANATIONS

1. **(B)** Consent is assumed from any patient requiring emergency intervention who is physically, mentally, or emotionally unable to provide expressed consent.

2. **(D)** Level III trauma center is the choice because it will stabilize and transfer serious patients as needed as part of a trauma system. Transport decisions will be dependent on many factors, one of those being transport time.

3. **(B)** Good Samaritan laws protect a paramedic if he or she acts in good faith and is not negligent, acts within his or her scope of practice, and does not accept payment for service.

4. **(B)** Vasopressin is indicated only for the management of ventricular fibrillation and pulseless ventricular tachycardia.

5. **(B)** Epinephrine 0.01 mg/kg of 1:10,000 solution is the recommended dose for pediatric cardiac arrest.

6. **(B)** A delayed hypersensitivity reaction may occur several hours or even days after exposure. Common causes are medications and chemicals. A patient may very well present with the signs/symptoms of allergic reaction several days after starting a new medication.

7. **(D)** This patient is alert and oriented, so he has an intact airway and is breathing. Your priority for this patient is "circulation," which includes stopping major hemorrhage. Applying a pressure dressing and elevation are necessary. **(A)** is incorrect because it is not a higher priority than controlling hemorrhage. **(B)** is not indicated for this patient. **(C)** is incorrect because it states right leg.

8. **(B)** A minimum of 100 compressions per minute. This is basic life support material you must be familiar with before taking your certification exam.

9. **(D)** A bag-valve mask device with a reservoir and an adequate oxygen source (at least 15 LPM) will deliver an oxygen concentration of 100%.

10. **(C)** A pulse oximetry reading of 90% in a person who is on high-flow oxygen indicates moderate hypoxia. Intubation should be considered.

11. **(B)** Excessive hyperventilation of a patient with increasing intracranial pressure can decrease the blood arterial carbon dioxide to dangerous levels.

12. **(D)** Decorticate posturing (flexion) indicates a lesion at or above the brain stem. Decerebrate posturing (extension) results from a lesion within the brain stem.

13. **(D)** 5 mg/kg of amiodarone is the recommended dose for the treatment of pulseless v tach or v fib in pediatric patients.

14. **(C)** Treatment for this unstable patient is synchronous cardioversion (since the patient has a pulse). If this patient was pulseless, the treatment would include defibrillation.

15. **(B)** Hyperventilation can result in an excess elimination of carbon dioxide leading to respiratory alkalosis.

16. **(B)** Beck's triad includes hypotension, distant heart tones, and JVD. This triad of symptoms can aid in the diagnosis of cardiac tamponade.

17. **(A)** Stridor is a harsh, high- or low-pitched sound caused by breathing through a partially blocked airway; wheezing **(B)** is a high- or low-pitched whistling sound; crackles/rhonchi **(C** and **D)** represent fluid/mucus in the larger bronchial airways.

18. **(B)** Murphy's sign is pain caused when an inflamed gallbladder is palpated by pressing under the right costal margin. McBurney's point **(A)** is a common site of pain from appendicitis located one to two inches above the anterior iliac crest in a direct line with the umbilicus. Grey-Turner's sign **(C)** is ecchymosis in the flank area. Cullen's sign **(D)** is ecchymosis in the periumbilical area.

19. **(B)** Demerol IV titrated for pain relief. **(A)** is incorrect; morphine is contraindicated because it is believed to cause spasm of the cystic duct in the gallbladder. **(C)** and **(D)** are incorrect because the dosages listed are wrong. Note: While there might be concern about use of pain medication in "undiagnosed" abdominal pain or the administration of pain medication may mask symptoms and make in-hospital assessment more difficult, the use of Demerol is not contraindicated in cholecystitis.

20. **(A)** Cushing's reflex includes an increase in systolic blood pressure, bradycardia, and erratic (usually slow) respirations.

21. **(D)** Lidocaine is contraindicated in severe degrees of SA, AV, or intraventricular blocks because it may produce serious ventricular dysrhythmias or develop into complete heart block.

22. **(C)** 30 compressions to 2 ventilations.

23. **(A)** Field extubation is not common. If it must be performed, the patient must clearly be able to maintain and protect his or her own airway and have adequate spontaneous respirations.

24. **(B)** Most newborn infants respond quite favorably to warming, drying, suctioning, and stimulation. Occasionally, administration of oxygen with assisted ventilations may be necessary. Vascular access and CPR are utilized only after the infant fails to respond effectively to ventilatory assistance.

25. **(D)** The three phases of the body's response to stress are alarm reaction (or the fight on flight response); resistance—as the body sustains increasing stress, the level of resistance to stress raises; therefore, higher levels of stress must occur for the alarm reaction to occur; exhaustion—as stress continues, coping mechanisms begin to fail.

26. **(C)** A pulse oximeter is used as an assessment tool. A patient with a pulse oximeter value of less than 90% with no apparent cause or past medical history is considered to be moderately hypoxic and needs high-flow oxygen administration.

27. **(D)** A history of taking birth control pills combined with signs and symptoms that include a painful and inflamed lower extremity suggest deep vein thrombosis. This predisposes the patient to developing a pulmonary embolus.

28. **(C)** This rhythm indicates atrial fibrillation with a rapid ventricular response.

29. **(A)** 100 times per minute.

30. **(C)** It is unclear if this patient fell, so you must suspect trauma and c-spine injury. A jaw-thrust maneuver and bag-valve mask ventilation is the best choice. **(A)** is incorrect because the oxygen flow setting is too low; it should be at least 15 LPM. **(B)** is incorrect because it utilizes a nonrebreather mask to assist ventilations; nonrebreathers are not designed for or capable of assisting ventilations. **(D)** is incorrect because the patient needs his ventilations assisted.

31. **(D)** Continued observation. The patient's vital signs do not indicate medication administration.

32. **(C)** Prearrival instructions provide immediate instructions and assistance to the caller prior to arrival of EMS units.

33. **(D)** The correct answer is all of the above. Chest pain and dysrhythmias are a typical sign/symptom of cocaine abuse. Confusion and polyuria represent alcohol use. Dilated pupils and anxiety are hallucinogens. Constricted pupils and respiratory depression are the result of opiates.

34. **(A)** The first medication to be delivered after defibrillating pulseless ventricular tachycardia is epinephrine or vasopressin.

35. **(A)** 0.5–1.0 joules/kg is the recommended energy setting when cardioversion is necessary. Repeat cardioversion can be increased to 2 joules/kg.

36. **(C)** Don't forget the basics! The head-tilt/chin-lift and jaw-thrust maneuver are both manual airway maneuvers that are very effective in initial management of the airway.

37. **(B)** A subdural hematoma is usually due to rupture of small venous vessels. This type of bleeding is slow and the onset of symptoms may take several hours to develop after the injury.

38. **(D)** Administration of nitroglycerin grⅠ/150 sublingual is the only correct choice for this question. Establishing an IV **(A)** is warranted for a patient complaining of chest pain but the IV should be run at KVO. Administration of Lasix **(B)** may be appropriate if signs/symptoms of left ventricular failure are present but the dose of 100 mg is excessive. You certainly want to administer oxygen **(C)** but a high-flow rate is recommended to increase oxygen delivery to the myocardium.

39. **(D)** The primary responsibility of the paramedic at all scenes is the protection of himself or herself and other EMS personnel.

40. **(B)** Supine hypotension syndrome (or vena cava syndrome) occurs when the pregnant uterus compresses the inferior vena cava when the patient is in a supine position. This results in a decrease in blood return back to the heart and a reduction of cardiac output. This syndrome can occur as early as the third month of gestation.

41. **(C)** The patient care report may be the only accurate account available to healthcare professionals, as well as other people interested in the event.

42. **(A)** This is a basic airway management question. The head-tilt/chin-lift maneuver is the simplest airway management technique to open the airway when no cervical spine trauma is suspected.

43. **(A)** The classic description of pain associated with a dissecting aortic aneurysm is a ripping or tearing sensation.

44. **(C)** Revisions are acceptable and must be done on a separate form and then attached to the original document.

45. **(C)** Transport for evaluation must be considered for this patient. A bradycardic rate of 48 while mowing the lawn on a hot August day should be a concern. With the presence of chest pain, you should suspect an underlying cardiac origin and transport.

46. **(D)** This rhythm is complete heart block. With the presence of serious signs/symptoms, immediate transcutaneous pacing is indicated.

47. **(C)** Treatment of seizure activity in eclampsia includes placing the patient in the left lateral recumbent position, maintaining the airway, administering high-flow oxygen, establishing IV access, and the administration of 2–5 grams of magnesium sulfate IV. If seizures cannot be controlled, sedatives may be required.

48. **(D)** In a tension pneumothorax, the patient is dealing with oxygenation problems and circulation problems. The tension pneumothorax creates an intrathoracic shift, impeding venous blood return to the heart.

49. **(C)** Both acids and alkalis cause burns by disrupting cell membranes and damaging tissues on contact. **(A)** is incorrect because antidotes and neutralizing agents should never be used as they may cause a violent reaction with the contaminant. **(B)** is incorrect because alkali burns are typically more severe because of their liquefaction necrosis process. **(D)** is incorrect because you should always approach from upwind.

50. **(C)** Procainamide should be discontinued if the QRS is widened 50% of its original width, the maximum dose is achieved, the arrhythmia is suppressed, or hypotension develops.

51. **(C)** Hyphema is a collection of blood in the anterior chamber of the eye due to trauma. This type of injury is a potential threat to the patient's vision and requires evaluation by an ophthalmologist.

52. **(D)** Right route. Amiodarone cannot be given via the endotracheal route. The six rights of medication administration include: right medication, right dose, right time, right route, right patient, and right documentation.

53. **(D)** Hyperthermia (fever) should not affect the accuracy of a pulse oximeter reading. Some circumstances that can affect accuracy include nail polish, acrylic nails, dark pigmentation or bruising, high bilirubin concentration.

54. **(C)** Prehospital indications for the administration of sodium bicarbonate include tricyclic antidepressant overdoses, hyperkalemia, and preexisting or suspected acidosis.

55. **(D)** Naloxone is used to reverse the effects of opiate toxicity. The recommended dose in pediatrics is 0.1 mg/kg.

56. **(C)** Applying gentle countertraction to the infant's head to prevent explosive delivery is essential to decrease the likelihood of tearing of the perineum and to decrease the potential for rapid expulsion of the baby's skull through the birth canal, which may cause intracranial injury.

57. **(A)** Adenocard is indicated for the treatment of a narrow complex tachycardia.

58. **(D)** Once every 6–8 seconds (8–10 breaths/minute).

59. **(D)** This ECG demonstrates a sinus tachycardia.

60. **(D)** Mechanism of injury can provide clues for determining possible injuries.

61. **(A)** CPR is indicated even if signs of death are present. A hypothermic patient cannot be presumed dead until a core body temperature of 94–95°F has been achieved and resuscitation efforts are still unsuccessful.

62. **(B)** Immediate defibrillation is required for this patient.

63. **(A)** IV medication may be administered, but spaced at longer than standard intervals; therefore **(C)** is incorrect. Drug metabolism is reduced so administered medication such as epinephrine and lidocaine may accumulate to toxic levels. In addition, administered drugs may remain in the peripheral circulation. When the patient is rewarmed and peripheral circulation resumes, a large toxic bolus of medication may be delivered to the central circulation. **(D)** is incorrect because lidocaine and procainamide will actually lower fibrillation threshold in a severely hypothermic patient. **(B)** is incorrect because medication should not be withheld unless the core temperature is below 86°F.

64. **(B)** The amount of energy required to deform a steering wheel is significant. Possible life-threatening injuries from the body striking a steering wheel include: flail chest, myocardial contusion, aortic tear, tracheal or vascular injuries, pulmonary contusion, pneumothorax, solid and hollow organ injury. Bilateral femur fractures may result if an "up-and-over" path occurred.

65. **(D)** Alcohol is a central nervous system depressant. Because of this, alcohol can mask signs and symptoms of injury. It is important to assess all trauma patients thoroughly, but be especially meticulous when you suspect drug/alcohol use.

66. **(A)** "Low-head" dams create a recirculating current, which can repeatedly pull the victim under the water, making escape difficult. These dams also make rescue operations hazardous.

67. **(C)** Making this patient a "load and go" patient based on the information provided is an inappropriate action.

68. **(D)** Inspiratory stridor, absence of drooling or trouble swallowing, and symptoms persistently worse at night, leads to the conclusion of the croup.

69. **(A)** An ectopic pregnancy should be suspected when abdominal pain is present in women of childbearing age who are sexually active. An ectopic pregnancy can be difficult to distinguish from other conditions. The classic triad of symptoms includes abdominal pain, vaginal bleeding, and amenorrhea. Other symptoms include referred pain to the shoulder, nausea, vomiting, or syncope. Signs of shock may be present if the ectopic ruptures.

70. **(D)** Inserting the needle over (on top of) the second or third rib avoids inadvertent puncturing or laceration of the adjoining vessels and nerves located at the inferior border of the ribs.

71. **(D)** Immediate transcutaneous pacing is indicated for Type Two second-degree AV block and third-degree AV block when accompanied with symptoms.

72. **(D)** Paroxysmal supraventricular tachycardia (PSVT) may require synchronized cardioversion, especially if the patient is hemodynamically unstable. Pulseless ventricular tachycardia and ventricular fibrillation require immediate defibrillation, not cardioversion.

73. **(B)** To correct an error on a PCR, a single line should be struck through the error with the EMT-paramedic's initials and date next to the error.

74. **(D)** Of the choices listed, oxygen is the only appropriate treatment. Nitroglycerin and aspirin are not indicated since the scenario does not include a complaint of chest pain.

75. **(A)** Long-term effects of hyperadrenalism lead to paper thin (almost transparent) skin that can be easily bruised or torn. The disease process also results in delayed healing, so great care with venipuncture is required. **(B)** is incorrect because IV therapy is *not* contraindicated. **(C)** is incorrect because you should never make an assumption about a patient's blood glucose level.

76. **(B)** Information related to the patient's condition or treatment is considered confidential information.

77. **(B)** Complications associated with a fracture of the clavicle include injury to the subclavian vein.

78. **(D)** When assessment of a trauma patient does not reveal significant injury, the presence of unexplained shock should lead you to suspect serious abdominal/thorax trauma.

79. **(D)** Respiratory failure, most probably due to pneumonia. This is based on tachypnea, increased work of breathing, diminished breath sounds, dullness to percussions, and elevated temperature.

80. **(B)** This patient has a valid DNR (Do Not Resuscitate) order and no obvious signs of life. The correct actions would be to address the survivor in terms that leave no doubt about the outcome of the deceased. Use gentle reassuring eye contact and offer any assistance that may be needed to the survivor.

81. **(B)** The nasopharyngeal airway should be measured from the tip of the nose to the earlobe.

82. **(C)** Heart rates ranging from 180 to 220 beats per minute in a child are considered SVT if the QRS complexes remain narrow. V tach presents with a wide QRS; sinus tachycardia usually shows P waves, and rapid atrial fibrillation will be irregularly irregular.

83. **(A)** During needle decompression, the needle is inserted on top of the third rib to ensure that the vein, artery, and nerve bundle under each rib are not damaged. Each intercostal space contains a vein, artery, and nerve, which lie *underneath* each rib.

84. **(C)** The patient's history should lead you to believe a vasovagal episode. Having a bowel movement or bearing down to have a bowel movement can stimulate the vagus nerve and slow down the heart rate enough to cause dizziness/syncope.

85. **(C)** Hypoglycemia is not considered an anginal equivalent.

86. **(D)** Defamation is intentional false communication that injures another person's reputation or good name. Defamation includes slander, which is verbal, and libel, which is written.

87. **(A)** With the probability of significant trauma and c-spine injury, the child's airway should be assessed using a jaw-thrust maneuver while stabilizing the cervical spine. Head-tilt/chin-lift hyperextension and hyperflexion (**B, C,** and **D**) cause manipulation of the cervical spine and are not indicated when cervical spine injury is suspected.

88. **(D)** This is a difficult question. If you knew this answer, pat yourself on the back. Brown-Sequard's syndrome is caused by a penetrating injury that affects one side of the spinal cord. The damage to the one side results in sensory and motor loss to that side of the body. Pain and temperature perception are lost on the opposite side of the body because of the switching of the associated nerves as they enter the spinal cord.

89. **(C)** Posterior pressure exerted on the cricoid cartilage (the Sellick maneuver) will effectively compress the esophagus, minimizing the potential for gastric distention. This maneuver will also reposition the vocal cords for clearer visualization of anatomic structures.

90. **(B)** The second dose of amiodarone for the treatment of ventricular fibrillation is 150 mg.

91. **(D)** Since it is unknown if there are any c-spine injuries from the fall through the ice, you must secure the airway and control the cervical spine during resuscitation.

92. **(C)** Nitroglycerin is a vasodilator; it works against vasospasm and decreases preload. It does not have an effect on afterload.

93. **(B)** Roles. Recognizing an emergency exists, assessing the situation, managing the emergency care, coordinating efforts of your team as well as other agencies involved in the care and transportation of the patient and establishing rapport with the patient and other EMS crew are all examples of a paramedic's roles.

94. **(B)** The first unit to arrive on the scene should begin the scene sizeup, which includes establishing command, calling for back-up units, controlling any hazards, and locating and triaging patients. It would not be appropriate for the primary unit to locate and transport the most critically injured patient.

95. **(D)** SLUDGE is a helpful mnemonic to remember signs of poisoning— S = salivation, L = lacrimation, U = urination, D = defecation, G = GI upset, E = emesis. Other symptoms of organophosphate poisoning include, bronchoconstriction, bradycardia, anxiety, and visual disturbances.

96. **(C)** One of the ways to determine successful placement of the IO needle is by aspiration of the bone marrow. Additionally, an unobstructed infusion of fluid without evidence of infiltration can also be used. X-rays are not needed to confirm placement. You should not be able to aspirate arterial blood from a properly placed IO needle.

97. **(A)** The safety officer monitors all on-scene actions to ensure that no potentially harmful situations are created.

98. **(C)** Place your hands on the lower half of the sternum at the nipple line.

99. **(B)** By the time the victim of a lightning strike is reached, the electricity will have dissipated. While you may be concerned as long as the storm remains nearby, there is no danger of electrical shock from touching the victim of a lightning strike.

100. **(C)** The recommended pediatric dose of diazepam is 0.1–0.3 mg/kg for the treatment of seizures.

101. **(C)** A flail chest is three or more adjacent ribs that are fractured in two or more places. This segment of the chest is free to move with the pressure changes of respirations.

102. **(C)** Paradoxical chest wall movement associated with flail chest is defined as the motion of a flail segment opposite to the normal motion of the chest wall.

103. **(C)** The signs and symptoms displayed by this patient are consistent with a left side tension pneumothorax and immediate chest decompression is required.

104. **(C)** The usual dose range of Compazine is 5–10 mg. It can be administered IV or IM.

105. **(D)** The signs and symptoms are consistent with a tension pneumothorax (absent breath sounds, tracheal deviation, no or little chest movement on the affected side). Immediate needle decompression is warranted.

106. **(A)** How fast the temperature of the child rises will increase a child's risk for developing a seizure. For example, a child who transitions from a temperature of 100.2 to 104.5°F in 30 minutes is more likely to suffer a febrile seizure than a child who develops a 104.5°F temperature over several hours.

107. **(B)** This patient was most likely intubated in the right mainstem bronchus. Deflating the endotracheal tube cuff, withdrawing the endotracheal tube slightly, reinflating the cuff, and reevaluating breath sounds is the proper procedure when a right mainstem bronchus intubation is suspected.

108. **(B)** 36% (chest = 9%, abdomen = 9%, entire arm 9%, front of the leg = 9%).

109. **(B)** Vasopressin is indicated in ventricular fibrillation at a dose of 40 units IV to be administered as a *one-time* dose.

110. **(A)** Abruptio placenta is premature separation of the placenta from the uterus. There are different presentations that can occur depending on the severity of the abruption. Classic presentation includes a sudden, sharp, tearing pain and the development of a stiff boardlike abdomen. Bleeding can be severe or not present depending on many factors.

111. **(C)** Abruptio placenta is premature separation of the placenta from the uterus and is a true medical emergency because it poses a life threat to the mother and fetus.

112. **(D)** Multigravida is when a woman has been pregnant more than once. Nullipara is a woman who has not yet delivered her first child. If you did not know this common terminology, you must review obstetric medical terminology.

113. (A) Valium (diazepam) is a sedative and anticonvulsant that depresses seizure activity in the brain. (C) and (D) are incorrect because the dose is wrong. (B) is not indicated with a blood glucose reading of 120 mg/dl.

114. (D) With the vital signs given in the scenario, the child is displaying signs and symptoms consistent with compensated shock. The shock is most probably related to diarrhea. A 20 cc/kg bolus of normal saline or an isotonic crystalloid fluid is recommended.

115. (C) The use of end-tidal carbon dioxide detection ($ETCO_2$) is one tool to assess for proper endotracheal tube placement. The absence of carbon dioxide likely indicates that the endotracheal tube has been placed in the esophagus. Verifying correct endotracheal tube placement is absolutely essential. $ETCO_2$ is only one method to assist in verification of proper placement.

116. (C) When using the rule of nines, the head of a child is assigned 18% BSA compared to 9% BSA on an adult. There are several other "rule of nine" modifications for children and infants you should be familiar with before taking your certification exam.

117. (C) Epiglottitis is a bacterial infection causing the acute swelling of the epiglottis and the soft tissues above the glottic opening. Clinical findings include but are not limited to: sudden onset high fever (102–105°F), pain on swallowing, typically sitting in tripod position, and drooling.

118. (C) Since the patient's presentation is considered stable, a vagal maneuver is indicated.

119. (B) Hypocalcemia results in decreased contractility and increased myocardial irritability. Hypomagnesemia results in increased myocardial irritability.

120. (B) An acute infarction to the inferior wall will present with ST segment elevation in leads II, III, and aVF. (D) is incorrect because ST segment depression indicates ischemia and not acute infarction.

Appendix

ADDITIONAL PRACTICE TEST ANSWER SHEETS

This appendix contains three additional answer sheets that can be used for the practice test in Chapter Eight.

Answer Sheet

PRACTICE TEST 1

1	Ⓐ Ⓑ Ⓒ Ⓓ	31	Ⓐ Ⓑ Ⓒ Ⓓ	61	Ⓐ Ⓑ Ⓒ Ⓓ	91	Ⓐ Ⓑ Ⓒ Ⓓ
2	Ⓐ Ⓑ Ⓒ Ⓓ	32	Ⓐ Ⓑ Ⓒ Ⓓ	62	Ⓐ Ⓑ Ⓒ Ⓓ	92	Ⓐ Ⓑ Ⓒ Ⓓ
3	Ⓐ Ⓑ Ⓒ Ⓓ	33	Ⓐ Ⓑ Ⓒ Ⓓ	63	Ⓐ Ⓑ Ⓒ Ⓓ	93	Ⓐ Ⓑ Ⓒ Ⓓ
4	Ⓐ Ⓑ Ⓒ Ⓓ	34	Ⓐ Ⓑ Ⓒ Ⓓ	64	Ⓐ Ⓑ Ⓒ Ⓓ	94	Ⓐ Ⓑ Ⓒ Ⓓ
5	Ⓐ Ⓑ Ⓒ Ⓓ	35	Ⓐ Ⓑ Ⓒ Ⓓ	65	Ⓐ Ⓑ Ⓒ Ⓓ	95	Ⓐ Ⓑ Ⓒ Ⓓ
6	Ⓐ Ⓑ Ⓒ Ⓓ	36	Ⓐ Ⓑ Ⓒ Ⓓ	66	Ⓐ Ⓑ Ⓒ Ⓓ	96	Ⓐ Ⓑ Ⓒ Ⓓ
7	Ⓐ Ⓑ Ⓒ Ⓓ	37	Ⓐ Ⓑ Ⓒ Ⓓ	67	Ⓐ Ⓑ Ⓒ Ⓓ	97	Ⓐ Ⓑ Ⓒ Ⓓ
8	Ⓐ Ⓑ Ⓒ Ⓓ	38	Ⓐ Ⓑ Ⓒ Ⓓ	68	Ⓐ Ⓑ Ⓒ Ⓓ	98	Ⓐ Ⓑ Ⓒ Ⓓ
9	Ⓐ Ⓑ Ⓒ Ⓓ	39	Ⓐ Ⓑ Ⓒ Ⓓ	69	Ⓐ Ⓑ Ⓒ Ⓓ	99	Ⓐ Ⓑ Ⓒ Ⓓ
10	Ⓐ Ⓑ Ⓒ Ⓓ	40	Ⓐ Ⓑ Ⓒ Ⓓ	70	Ⓐ Ⓑ Ⓒ Ⓓ	100	Ⓐ Ⓑ Ⓒ Ⓓ
11	Ⓐ Ⓑ Ⓒ Ⓓ	41	Ⓐ Ⓑ Ⓒ Ⓓ	71	Ⓐ Ⓑ Ⓒ Ⓓ	101	Ⓐ Ⓑ Ⓒ Ⓓ
12	Ⓐ Ⓑ Ⓒ Ⓓ	42	Ⓐ Ⓑ Ⓒ Ⓓ	72	Ⓐ Ⓑ Ⓒ Ⓓ	102	Ⓐ Ⓑ Ⓒ Ⓓ
13	Ⓐ Ⓑ Ⓒ Ⓓ	43	Ⓐ Ⓑ Ⓒ Ⓓ	73	Ⓐ Ⓑ Ⓒ Ⓓ	103	Ⓐ Ⓑ Ⓒ Ⓓ
14	Ⓐ Ⓑ Ⓒ Ⓓ	44	Ⓐ Ⓑ Ⓒ Ⓓ	74	Ⓐ Ⓑ Ⓒ Ⓓ	104	Ⓐ Ⓑ Ⓒ Ⓓ
15	Ⓐ Ⓑ Ⓒ Ⓓ	45	Ⓐ Ⓑ Ⓒ Ⓓ	75	Ⓐ Ⓑ Ⓒ Ⓓ	105	Ⓐ Ⓑ Ⓒ Ⓓ
16	Ⓐ Ⓑ Ⓒ Ⓓ	46	Ⓐ Ⓑ Ⓒ Ⓓ	76	Ⓐ Ⓑ Ⓒ Ⓓ	106	Ⓐ Ⓑ Ⓒ Ⓓ
17	Ⓐ Ⓑ Ⓒ Ⓓ	47	Ⓐ Ⓑ Ⓒ Ⓓ	77	Ⓐ Ⓑ Ⓒ Ⓓ	107	Ⓐ Ⓑ Ⓒ Ⓓ
18	Ⓐ Ⓑ Ⓒ Ⓓ	48	Ⓐ Ⓑ Ⓒ Ⓓ	78	Ⓐ Ⓑ Ⓒ Ⓓ	108	Ⓐ Ⓑ Ⓒ Ⓓ
19	Ⓐ Ⓑ Ⓒ Ⓓ	49	Ⓐ Ⓑ Ⓒ Ⓓ	79	Ⓐ Ⓑ Ⓒ Ⓓ	109	Ⓐ Ⓑ Ⓒ Ⓓ
20	Ⓐ Ⓑ Ⓒ Ⓓ	50	Ⓐ Ⓑ Ⓒ Ⓓ	80	Ⓐ Ⓑ Ⓒ Ⓓ	110	Ⓐ Ⓑ Ⓒ Ⓓ
21	Ⓐ Ⓑ Ⓒ Ⓓ	51	Ⓐ Ⓑ Ⓒ Ⓓ	81	Ⓐ Ⓑ Ⓒ Ⓓ	111	Ⓐ Ⓑ Ⓒ Ⓓ
22	Ⓐ Ⓑ Ⓒ Ⓓ	52	Ⓐ Ⓑ Ⓒ Ⓓ	82	Ⓐ Ⓑ Ⓒ Ⓓ	112	Ⓐ Ⓑ Ⓒ Ⓓ
23	Ⓐ Ⓑ Ⓒ Ⓓ	53	Ⓐ Ⓑ Ⓒ Ⓓ	83	Ⓐ Ⓑ Ⓒ Ⓓ	113	Ⓐ Ⓑ Ⓒ Ⓓ
24	Ⓐ Ⓑ Ⓒ Ⓓ	54	Ⓐ Ⓑ Ⓒ Ⓓ	84	Ⓐ Ⓑ Ⓒ Ⓓ	114	Ⓐ Ⓑ Ⓒ Ⓓ
25	Ⓐ Ⓑ Ⓒ Ⓓ	55	Ⓐ Ⓑ Ⓒ Ⓓ	85	Ⓐ Ⓑ Ⓒ Ⓓ	115	Ⓐ Ⓑ Ⓒ Ⓓ
26	Ⓐ Ⓑ Ⓒ Ⓓ	56	Ⓐ Ⓑ Ⓒ Ⓓ	86	Ⓐ Ⓑ Ⓒ Ⓓ	116	Ⓐ Ⓑ Ⓒ Ⓓ
27	Ⓐ Ⓑ Ⓒ Ⓓ	57	Ⓐ Ⓑ Ⓒ Ⓓ	87	Ⓐ Ⓑ Ⓒ Ⓓ	117	Ⓐ Ⓑ Ⓒ Ⓓ
28	Ⓐ Ⓑ Ⓒ Ⓓ	58	Ⓐ Ⓑ Ⓒ Ⓓ	88	Ⓐ Ⓑ Ⓒ Ⓓ	118	Ⓐ Ⓑ Ⓒ Ⓓ
29	Ⓐ Ⓑ Ⓒ Ⓓ	59	Ⓐ Ⓑ Ⓒ Ⓓ	89	Ⓐ Ⓑ Ⓒ Ⓓ	119	Ⓐ Ⓑ Ⓒ Ⓓ
30	Ⓐ Ⓑ Ⓒ Ⓓ	60	Ⓐ Ⓑ Ⓒ Ⓓ	90	Ⓐ Ⓑ Ⓒ Ⓓ	120	Ⓐ Ⓑ Ⓒ Ⓓ

Answer Sheet

PRACTICE TEST 1

1 Ⓐ Ⓑ Ⓒ Ⓓ	31 Ⓐ Ⓑ Ⓒ Ⓓ	61 Ⓐ Ⓑ Ⓒ Ⓓ	91 Ⓐ Ⓑ Ⓒ Ⓓ
2 Ⓐ Ⓑ Ⓒ Ⓓ	32 Ⓐ Ⓑ Ⓒ Ⓓ	62 Ⓐ Ⓑ Ⓒ Ⓓ	92 Ⓐ Ⓑ Ⓒ Ⓓ
3 Ⓐ Ⓑ Ⓒ Ⓓ	33 Ⓐ Ⓑ Ⓒ Ⓓ	63 Ⓐ Ⓑ Ⓒ Ⓓ	93 Ⓐ Ⓑ Ⓒ Ⓓ
4 Ⓐ Ⓑ Ⓒ Ⓓ	34 Ⓐ Ⓑ Ⓒ Ⓓ	64 Ⓐ Ⓑ Ⓒ Ⓓ	94 Ⓐ Ⓑ Ⓒ Ⓓ
5 Ⓐ Ⓑ Ⓒ Ⓓ	35 Ⓐ Ⓑ Ⓒ Ⓓ	65 Ⓐ Ⓑ Ⓒ Ⓓ	95 Ⓐ Ⓑ Ⓒ Ⓓ
6 Ⓐ Ⓑ Ⓒ Ⓓ	36 Ⓐ Ⓑ Ⓒ Ⓓ	66 Ⓐ Ⓑ Ⓒ Ⓓ	96 Ⓐ Ⓑ Ⓒ Ⓓ
7 Ⓐ Ⓑ Ⓒ Ⓓ	37 Ⓐ Ⓑ Ⓒ Ⓓ	67 Ⓐ Ⓑ Ⓒ Ⓓ	97 Ⓐ Ⓑ Ⓒ Ⓓ
8 Ⓐ Ⓑ Ⓒ Ⓓ	38 Ⓐ Ⓑ Ⓒ Ⓓ	68 Ⓐ Ⓑ Ⓒ Ⓓ	98 Ⓐ Ⓑ Ⓒ Ⓓ
9 Ⓐ Ⓑ Ⓒ Ⓓ	39 Ⓐ Ⓑ Ⓒ Ⓓ	69 Ⓐ Ⓑ Ⓒ Ⓓ	99 Ⓐ Ⓑ Ⓒ Ⓓ
10 Ⓐ Ⓑ Ⓒ Ⓓ	40 Ⓐ Ⓑ Ⓒ Ⓓ	70 Ⓐ Ⓑ Ⓒ Ⓓ	100 Ⓐ Ⓑ Ⓒ Ⓓ
11 Ⓐ Ⓑ Ⓒ Ⓓ	41 Ⓐ Ⓑ Ⓒ Ⓓ	71 Ⓐ Ⓑ Ⓒ Ⓓ	101 Ⓐ Ⓑ Ⓒ Ⓓ
12 Ⓐ Ⓑ Ⓒ Ⓓ	42 Ⓐ Ⓑ Ⓒ Ⓓ	72 Ⓐ Ⓑ Ⓒ Ⓓ	102 Ⓐ Ⓑ Ⓒ Ⓓ
13 Ⓐ Ⓑ Ⓒ Ⓓ	43 Ⓐ Ⓑ Ⓒ Ⓓ	73 Ⓐ Ⓑ Ⓒ Ⓓ	103 Ⓐ Ⓑ Ⓒ Ⓓ
14 Ⓐ Ⓑ Ⓒ Ⓓ	44 Ⓐ Ⓑ Ⓒ Ⓓ	74 Ⓐ Ⓑ Ⓒ Ⓓ	104 Ⓐ Ⓑ Ⓒ Ⓓ
15 Ⓐ Ⓑ Ⓒ Ⓓ	45 Ⓐ Ⓑ Ⓒ Ⓓ	75 Ⓐ Ⓑ Ⓒ Ⓓ	105 Ⓐ Ⓑ Ⓒ Ⓓ
16 Ⓐ Ⓑ Ⓒ Ⓓ	46 Ⓐ Ⓑ Ⓒ Ⓓ	76 Ⓐ Ⓑ Ⓒ Ⓓ	106 Ⓐ Ⓑ Ⓒ Ⓓ
17 Ⓐ Ⓑ Ⓒ Ⓓ	47 Ⓐ Ⓑ Ⓒ Ⓓ	77 Ⓐ Ⓑ Ⓒ Ⓓ	107 Ⓐ Ⓑ Ⓒ Ⓓ
18 Ⓐ Ⓑ Ⓒ Ⓓ	48 Ⓐ Ⓑ Ⓒ Ⓓ	78 Ⓐ Ⓑ Ⓒ Ⓓ	108 Ⓐ Ⓑ Ⓒ Ⓓ
19 Ⓐ Ⓑ Ⓒ Ⓓ	49 Ⓐ Ⓑ Ⓒ Ⓓ	79 Ⓐ Ⓑ Ⓒ Ⓓ	109 Ⓐ Ⓑ Ⓒ Ⓓ
20 Ⓐ Ⓑ Ⓒ Ⓓ	50 Ⓐ Ⓑ Ⓒ Ⓓ	80 Ⓐ Ⓑ Ⓒ Ⓓ	110 Ⓐ Ⓑ Ⓒ Ⓓ
21 Ⓐ Ⓑ Ⓒ Ⓓ	51 Ⓐ Ⓑ Ⓒ Ⓓ	81 Ⓐ Ⓑ Ⓒ Ⓓ	111 Ⓐ Ⓑ Ⓒ Ⓓ
22 Ⓐ Ⓑ Ⓒ Ⓓ	52 Ⓐ Ⓑ Ⓒ Ⓓ	82 Ⓐ Ⓑ Ⓒ Ⓓ	112 Ⓐ Ⓑ Ⓒ Ⓓ
23 Ⓐ Ⓑ Ⓒ Ⓓ	53 Ⓐ Ⓑ Ⓒ Ⓓ	83 Ⓐ Ⓑ Ⓒ Ⓓ	113 Ⓐ Ⓑ Ⓒ Ⓓ
24 Ⓐ Ⓑ Ⓒ Ⓓ	54 Ⓐ Ⓑ Ⓒ Ⓓ	84 Ⓐ Ⓑ Ⓒ Ⓓ	114 Ⓐ Ⓑ Ⓒ Ⓓ
25 Ⓐ Ⓑ Ⓒ Ⓓ	55 Ⓐ Ⓑ Ⓒ Ⓓ	85 Ⓐ Ⓑ Ⓒ Ⓓ	115 Ⓐ Ⓑ Ⓒ Ⓓ
26 Ⓐ Ⓑ Ⓒ Ⓓ	56 Ⓐ Ⓑ Ⓒ Ⓓ	86 Ⓐ Ⓑ Ⓒ Ⓓ	116 Ⓐ Ⓑ Ⓒ Ⓓ
27 Ⓐ Ⓑ Ⓒ Ⓓ	57 Ⓐ Ⓑ Ⓒ Ⓓ	87 Ⓐ Ⓑ Ⓒ Ⓓ	117 Ⓐ Ⓑ Ⓒ Ⓓ
28 Ⓐ Ⓑ Ⓒ Ⓓ	58 Ⓐ Ⓑ Ⓒ Ⓓ	88 Ⓐ Ⓑ Ⓒ Ⓓ	118 Ⓐ Ⓑ Ⓒ Ⓓ
29 Ⓐ Ⓑ Ⓒ Ⓓ	59 Ⓐ Ⓑ Ⓒ Ⓓ	89 Ⓐ Ⓑ Ⓒ Ⓓ	119 Ⓐ Ⓑ Ⓒ Ⓓ
30 Ⓐ Ⓑ Ⓒ Ⓓ	60 Ⓐ Ⓑ Ⓒ Ⓓ	90 Ⓐ Ⓑ Ⓒ Ⓓ	120 Ⓐ Ⓑ Ⓒ Ⓓ

Answer Sheet

PRACTICE TEST 1

1 Ⓐ Ⓑ Ⓒ Ⓓ	31 Ⓐ Ⓑ Ⓒ Ⓓ	61 Ⓐ Ⓑ Ⓒ Ⓓ	91 Ⓐ Ⓑ Ⓒ Ⓓ
2 Ⓐ Ⓑ Ⓒ Ⓓ	32 Ⓐ Ⓑ Ⓒ Ⓓ	62 Ⓐ Ⓑ Ⓒ Ⓓ	92 Ⓐ Ⓑ Ⓒ Ⓓ
3 Ⓐ Ⓑ Ⓒ Ⓓ	33 Ⓐ Ⓑ Ⓒ Ⓓ	63 Ⓐ Ⓑ Ⓒ Ⓓ	93 Ⓐ Ⓑ Ⓒ Ⓓ
4 Ⓐ Ⓑ Ⓒ Ⓓ	34 Ⓐ Ⓑ Ⓒ Ⓓ	64 Ⓐ Ⓑ Ⓒ Ⓓ	94 Ⓐ Ⓑ Ⓒ Ⓓ
5 Ⓐ Ⓑ Ⓒ Ⓓ	35 Ⓐ Ⓑ Ⓒ Ⓓ	65 Ⓐ Ⓑ Ⓒ Ⓓ	95 Ⓐ Ⓑ Ⓒ Ⓓ
6 Ⓐ Ⓑ Ⓒ Ⓓ	36 Ⓐ Ⓑ Ⓒ Ⓓ	66 Ⓐ Ⓑ Ⓒ Ⓓ	96 Ⓐ Ⓑ Ⓒ Ⓓ
7 Ⓐ Ⓑ Ⓒ Ⓓ	37 Ⓐ Ⓑ Ⓒ Ⓓ	67 Ⓐ Ⓑ Ⓒ Ⓓ	97 Ⓐ Ⓑ Ⓒ Ⓓ
8 Ⓐ Ⓑ Ⓒ Ⓓ	38 Ⓐ Ⓑ Ⓒ Ⓓ	68 Ⓐ Ⓑ Ⓒ Ⓓ	98 Ⓐ Ⓑ Ⓒ Ⓓ
9 Ⓐ Ⓑ Ⓒ Ⓓ	39 Ⓐ Ⓑ Ⓒ Ⓓ	69 Ⓐ Ⓑ Ⓒ Ⓓ	99 Ⓐ Ⓑ Ⓒ Ⓓ
10 Ⓐ Ⓑ Ⓒ Ⓓ	40 Ⓐ Ⓑ Ⓒ Ⓓ	70 Ⓐ Ⓑ Ⓒ Ⓓ	100 Ⓐ Ⓑ Ⓒ Ⓓ
11 Ⓐ Ⓑ Ⓒ Ⓓ	41 Ⓐ Ⓑ Ⓒ Ⓓ	71 Ⓐ Ⓑ Ⓒ Ⓓ	101 Ⓐ Ⓑ Ⓒ Ⓓ
12 Ⓐ Ⓑ Ⓒ Ⓓ	42 Ⓐ Ⓑ Ⓒ Ⓓ	72 Ⓐ Ⓑ Ⓒ Ⓓ	102 Ⓐ Ⓑ Ⓒ Ⓓ
13 Ⓐ Ⓑ Ⓒ Ⓓ	43 Ⓐ Ⓑ Ⓒ Ⓓ	73 Ⓐ Ⓑ Ⓒ Ⓓ	103 Ⓐ Ⓑ Ⓒ Ⓓ
14 Ⓐ Ⓑ Ⓒ Ⓓ	44 Ⓐ Ⓑ Ⓒ Ⓓ	74 Ⓐ Ⓑ Ⓒ Ⓓ	104 Ⓐ Ⓑ Ⓒ Ⓓ
15 Ⓐ Ⓑ Ⓒ Ⓓ	45 Ⓐ Ⓑ Ⓒ Ⓓ	75 Ⓐ Ⓑ Ⓒ Ⓓ	105 Ⓐ Ⓑ Ⓒ Ⓓ
16 Ⓐ Ⓑ Ⓒ Ⓓ	46 Ⓐ Ⓑ Ⓒ Ⓓ	76 Ⓐ Ⓑ Ⓒ Ⓓ	106 Ⓐ Ⓑ Ⓒ Ⓓ
17 Ⓐ Ⓑ Ⓒ Ⓓ	47 Ⓐ Ⓑ Ⓒ Ⓓ	77 Ⓐ Ⓑ Ⓒ Ⓓ	107 Ⓐ Ⓑ Ⓒ Ⓓ
18 Ⓐ Ⓑ Ⓒ Ⓓ	48 Ⓐ Ⓑ Ⓒ Ⓓ	78 Ⓐ Ⓑ Ⓒ Ⓓ	108 Ⓐ Ⓑ Ⓒ Ⓓ
19 Ⓐ Ⓑ Ⓒ Ⓓ	49 Ⓐ Ⓑ Ⓒ Ⓓ	79 Ⓐ Ⓑ Ⓒ Ⓓ	109 Ⓐ Ⓑ Ⓒ Ⓓ
20 Ⓐ Ⓑ Ⓒ Ⓓ	50 Ⓐ Ⓑ Ⓒ Ⓓ	80 Ⓐ Ⓑ Ⓒ Ⓓ	110 Ⓐ Ⓑ Ⓒ Ⓓ
21 Ⓐ Ⓑ Ⓒ Ⓓ	51 Ⓐ Ⓑ Ⓒ Ⓓ	81 Ⓐ Ⓑ Ⓒ Ⓓ	111 Ⓐ Ⓑ Ⓒ Ⓓ
22 Ⓐ Ⓑ Ⓒ Ⓓ	52 Ⓐ Ⓑ Ⓒ Ⓓ	82 Ⓐ Ⓑ Ⓒ Ⓓ	112 Ⓐ Ⓑ Ⓒ Ⓓ
23 Ⓐ Ⓑ Ⓒ Ⓓ	53 Ⓐ Ⓑ Ⓒ Ⓓ	83 Ⓐ Ⓑ Ⓒ Ⓓ	113 Ⓐ Ⓑ Ⓒ Ⓓ
24 Ⓐ Ⓑ Ⓒ Ⓓ	54 Ⓐ Ⓑ Ⓒ Ⓓ	84 Ⓐ Ⓑ Ⓒ Ⓓ	114 Ⓐ Ⓑ Ⓒ Ⓓ
25 Ⓐ Ⓑ Ⓒ Ⓓ	55 Ⓐ Ⓑ Ⓒ Ⓓ	85 Ⓐ Ⓑ Ⓒ Ⓓ	115 Ⓐ Ⓑ Ⓒ Ⓓ
26 Ⓐ Ⓑ Ⓒ Ⓓ	56 Ⓐ Ⓑ Ⓒ Ⓓ	86 Ⓐ Ⓑ Ⓒ Ⓓ	116 Ⓐ Ⓑ Ⓒ Ⓓ
27 Ⓐ Ⓑ Ⓒ Ⓓ	57 Ⓐ Ⓑ Ⓒ Ⓓ	87 Ⓐ Ⓑ Ⓒ Ⓓ	117 Ⓐ Ⓑ Ⓒ Ⓓ
28 Ⓐ Ⓑ Ⓒ Ⓓ	58 Ⓐ Ⓑ Ⓒ Ⓓ	88 Ⓐ Ⓑ Ⓒ Ⓓ	118 Ⓐ Ⓑ Ⓒ Ⓓ
29 Ⓐ Ⓑ Ⓒ Ⓓ	59 Ⓐ Ⓑ Ⓒ Ⓓ	89 Ⓐ Ⓑ Ⓒ Ⓓ	119 Ⓐ Ⓑ Ⓒ Ⓓ
30 Ⓐ Ⓑ Ⓒ Ⓓ	60 Ⓐ Ⓑ Ⓒ Ⓓ	90 Ⓐ Ⓑ Ⓒ Ⓓ	120 Ⓐ Ⓑ Ⓒ Ⓓ